ABOUT THE AUTHOR

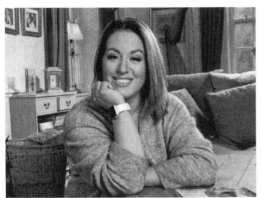

Meet Kate Grosvenor – a life coach, motivational speaker, best-selling author, and the woman behind the transformative *UncompliKated Perimenopause Series (guide, workbook, journal & diary).*

Once in her early 40s, Kate found herself facing a life that felt more like a labyrinth than a path. Fuelled by the determination to shape a brighter future for herself and her three daughters, she made the life-altering decision to climb out of the darkness. Leveraging her background in psychology, Kate dived deep into a plethora of resources – from books and seminars to podcasts and videos – making her own revival her full-time job.

Why does Kate do what she does? Because she knows she's not alone. She's made it her mission to ensure no woman has to reach the lows she once encountered. Since her climb back to a more fulfilling life, Kate has successfully coached thousands of women around the world, offering 1-2-1 coaching, group programmes, and eye-opening workshops.

Kate is not just a life coach; she's a perimenopause warrior herself. Misdiagnosed multiple times in her early 40s, Kate decided that the confusing journey to understanding perimenopause should be made easier for others. So, she committed to raising awareness and has been helping women globally ever since.

Her TikTok and YouTube videos have reached millions around the world on the topic of Perimenopause so writing a book seemed like another way to reach more women about this often-overlooked topic.

But Kate's life isn't all seminars and coaching calls. She's the proud mum to three daughters and two stepdaughters, aged 16-24. She and her partner share their quirky, much-loved (and occasionally falling apart) old home with a lively household of six cats and three horses. There's rarely a dull moment in the household!

Ready to turn the page? Kate is here to guide you through your perimenopause journey, offering not just professional expertise but also a hearty dose of real-world experience and warm encouragement. Let Kate help you navigate the maze of perimenopause. You're not alone; you're in compassionate, experienced hands.

Copyright

Title: The UncompliKated Guide to Perimenopause

First published in Great Britain in 2023

Address Epic House, 18 Darnall Road, Sheffield, S9 5AB. United Kingdom

Book design: Kate Grosvenor

Editing: Paul Hunt

Author Photograph: Collette Evans

While the author has taken great care to present accurate and current information at the time this book was published, it's important to note that medical science is ever evolving. Because of this and the unique variables that come with individual circumstances, readers are strongly advised to consult with a qualified healthcare provide for personalised guidance. This book should not serve as a substitute for professional medical advice, which should always be sought prior to making any health-related decisions. The author disclaims any liability for inaccuracy or omissions in this text and cannot be held accountable for any actions taken based on the information herein. Any reliance on this material is solely at the reader's own risk.

With huge thanks to all the women who have talked to me about their perimenopause journeys, my wonderful Da for editing and proofreading this text, my amazing and supportive partner, Scott, who helps me to dare to jump, and my girls, Gabriella, Rowan and Jenna, for being their fabulous selves.

THE
UNCOMPLIKATED
GUIDE TO
PERIMENOPAUSE

Kate Grosvenor

To All the Brave Women Navigating Perimenopause,
This book is for you – the unsung heroines facing hot flushes and hormone havoc with grace and grit. May you find guidance, affirmation, and a touch of humour in these pages.

TABLE OF CONTENTS

About the Author   1

Chapter 1 The Ups, Downs, and Roundabouts   9

Chapter 2 Peri-What-Now?   15

Chapter 3 The Hormonal Hokey Cokey   18

Chapter 4 Perimenopause Symptoms   27

Chapter 5 The Perimenopause Puzzle   37

Chapter 6 From Stress Fest to Zen Zone   45

Chapter 7 Be Still My Beating heart   51

Chapter 8 Dem Bones, Dem Bones, Dem Not-So-Dry Bones   56

Chapter 9 Where Did I Put My Keys?   60

Chapter 10 Thunderbolts and Lightning, Very, Very Frightening?   71

Chapter 11 Your Overflowing Bath and How to Plug It   80

Chapter 12 Tummy Troubles and Hormonal Hubbub   84

Chapter 13 The Softening Edges   97

Chapter 14 The Vagina Monologue   110

Chapter 15 The Ebb and Flow Reimagined   118

Chapter 16 Mental Health Matters   123

Chapter 17 Love in the Time of Hormones   135

Chapter 18 Beauty and the Hormonal Best   147

Chapter 19 No Snooze, You Lose   158

Chapter 20 Feeling Creaky?   175

Chapter 21 Hot Flushes & Cold Truths   183

Chapter 22 Ear We Go Again!   191

Chapter 23 The Perimenopausal Potpourri   203

Chapter 24 HRT Backstage Pass   232

Chapter 25 Level 1 of Healing Top of Form   239

Chapter 26 Stand Up and Be Counted   257

Chapter 27 Healing Level 2   265

Chapter 28 Healing Level 3   277

Chapter 29 Healing Level 4   297

Chapter 30 Recommended Supplements for Perimenopause   312

Chapter 31 The Journey Ahead   320

Chapter 32 Perimenopause Glossary of Terms   324

Chapter 33 Useful Resources   340

Index   342

Chapter 1:
THE UPS, DOWNS,
AND ROUNDABOUTS

My perimenopause journey that sparked this guide

In my mid-forties, I found that my body just kept going a bit 'wonky.' My first memory of something feeling wrong was around 44 (although in hindsight some of the weird ear-related dizziness phases could have also been a perimenopause thing). It all started with dizziness and brand-new allergies, and an all-encompassing feeling of nausea – almost like morning-sickness, so I bizarrely thought it might be pregnancy. It wasn't. But I just couldn't explain it.

Then I developed a strange rash on my face. Then an itchy ear. Then my headaches got worse. Then tiredness started to get overwhelming. I went back to the GPs again and again, and to be honest, they were lovely. However, they couldn't find out what was wrong, and they tested me for so many things . . . complete blood works, random viral things, and couldn't find anything abnormal. And so, my symptoms continued.

By the age of 45, I wondered if it could be hormonal, but I was told I was far too young for 'all of that'!

And so, at the ripe old age of 47, it got so bad that I couldn't enjoy a day out without the nausea making me feel like I was on a boat way out at sea, and the fatigue like I was only half-alive. It was at that point that I started researching what it could be. As a life coach, I speak to women all day every day, and there was a distinct pattern emerging.

So instead of seeing a GP (no offence to all the lovely doctors out there) I went to see a senior nurse practitioner, a woman of my own age. As soon as we started talking, she nodded along with everything I was saying, and agreed that there was a very real chance it was hormonal – the one test that I had been refused over and over again. And because I was over the age of 45 there was no need for a blood test. She listened to my symptoms and prescribed HRT for me there and then.

I already had the Mirena coil, which was giving me progesterone, so for oestrogen, given that there was a national shortage of gel at the time (don't get me started about that subject) I was given tablets. I would so love to tell you that it was all rainbows and roses, and it was the magic fix. It wasn't. It made me feel truly horrible and I stopped taking them after a few weeks.

I have never been a quitter. I went back and asked for another option and was given the patch instead. Halleluiah, that was better! And it was then that I realised that this topic was even more complicated, intricate, and personal than I had thought.

MacBook in hand, I started my research and went down a gazillion rabbit holes before the truth started to emerge: this was something that would (and does) affect all women. The menopause (not even perimenopause) that was barely discussed in my own parents' generation (often called 'the change') was not this. This was a longer journey, a more complicated, more diverse journey, and there was so much mystery, lack of information, no discussion, and even shame, around the topic.

Perimenopause, as I discovered, was the important chapter. Menopause itself is only one day in time (a year since your last period). In contrast perimenopause is, on average, ten years, but could be up to fifteen.

To put this in perspective, your teenage years are only seven years, and remember the angst there? Add a few more years on, and then add on all the multi-tasking, multiple responsibilities, feeling dead inside, dealing with children and/or ageing parents, more responsibility at work, and the fact that few or no allowances are made for you, and that there isn't much awareness of the symptoms, and you are part way to understanding the perimenopause and the effect it has on your life.

The good news is that you're not alone! Women are starting the conversation, banging our proverbial drum, and putting perimenopause on the map. That's why I wrote this book, why I have a support group on Facebook, why I talk about it every day on TikTok, etc. We *need* to have the word out there, shouting it loud and proud from the rooftops.

So here we are, a few years later, after hundreds of conversations with women all around the world, with a book which I hope you will find to be your most-treasured handbook through this chapter of your life.

It's the information I wish I had known, and the answers to the questions I get asked every day. I hope it gives you all of the knowledge that allows you to make informed decisions about your body, your mental health, and your life, and is your go-to guide from thousands of women who have been on the journey too.

First on the agenda is decoding the hormonal shifts that accompany perimenopause. In simple terms, I'm going to delve into what makes your body tick differently during this period. I'll be diving deep but keeping it jargon-free as much as I can, allowing you to truly grasp the biological underpinnings of what you're going through. After all, knowledge is power, and we're empowering you to understand this phase from the cellular level up.

I'll also help you to navigate the maze of healing options, including hormone replacement therapy (HRT). I'll go through the pros and cons, helping you to make an informed decision tailored to your unique circumstances.

I'll be offering you first-hand experience. Expect practical, real-world advice that speaks directly to you, no matter where you are on your journey. I've also listened to hundreds of women's stories in my coaching practice, so rest assured, you're in good hands.

I've also compiled a supplement guide for you. With endless products on the market, each promising the elixir of youth or the balm for every ache, it's hard to discern which ones can genuinely benefit you. My ultimate supplements guide cuts through the clutter, offering transparent, evidence-based advice.

Life is better with a bit of humour, isn't it? Throughout the book, you'll find real-life anecdotes that add levity to the subject. While perimenopause is a serious life stage, a dash of humour can make the journey more enjoyable and relatable.

Finally, for those who find medical terminology to be a bit like reading a foreign language, I have a glossary waiting for you at the end of this book. You'll never be lost in the jargon, empowering you to converse confidently about this topic whether it's with your GP or during a coffee catch-up with friends.

So, are you ready to reclaim the driver's seat of your well-being? By the end of this book, you'll not only understand the perimenopausal changes occurring in your body but also arm yourself with actionable advice. You'll be ready to tackle this life chapter like the well-seasoned, incredible woman you are.

It may be of interest to you that I have also written a few accompanying books/resources that work seamlessly with this guide— it's like your comprehensive toolkit for navigating one of life's most transformative phases with grace and confidence. Each component of this four-part series offers a unique blend of expert advice, actionable insights, and compassionate guidance to help you not just survive, but thrive through perimenopause. Here is a brief explanation of each:

1. **The UncompliKated Guide to Perimenopause**: This cornerstone book lays the foundation, providing an in-depth look at what perimenopause is, hormonal changes, and an array of healing options. It's the definitive guide that every woman should read to understand what's happening to her body.

2. **The UncompliKated Perimenopause Workbook**: This hands-on workbook dives into practical exercises involving CBT, self-compassion, and self-care. With daily and weekly trackers, you can measure your progress and set the course for happier, healthier days ahead.

3. **The UncompliKated Perimenopause Journal**: An intimate space for you to jot down your thoughts, symptoms, and feelings. This journal is perfect for self-reflection and serves as a helpful log when discussing symptoms with your healthcare provider.

4. **The UncompliKated Perimenopause Diary**: Plan your days while keeping track of symptoms, appointments, and self-care activities. This diary is a lifesaver for staying organised and balanced during this tumultuous time.

This series embodies my coaching philosophy, which combines evidence-based techniques, lived experiences, and a dash of humour. Whether you're at the start of your perimenopause journey or knee-deep in hot flushes, the "UncompliKated Perimenopause Series" is your ultimate companion for stepping into this new chapter with empowerment and ease.

Let's turn the page and get started, shall we? I hope you find this book invaluable, and you get all the answers you're looking for.

It's written with buckets full of love, from me to you.

Kate x

Chapter 2

PERI-WHAT-NOW?

Decoding the enigma of perimenopause

Ah, perimenopause: it's like puberty's older, wiser, yet somehow even more complicated sibling, isn't it?

First things first, let's clear the air. Perimenopause is not menopause. Think of it as the prelude, the opening act, or even the red carpet before the main event of menopause. While menopause is a single point in time – defined precisely as one year after your final menstrual period –perimenopause is the transitional phase leading up to that point.

It's kind of like that relative who arrives at the party way before it starts and leaves way after it's finished. It might linger for five months or set up camp for fifteen years; basically, it has no concept of time! You see, every woman's journey here is a custom-designed, special edition. You could be embracing this phase as early as your late 30s, early 40s or maybe sending out invitations at 51; it's a "you-do-you" situation, ladies.

So, in a nutshell, perimenopause is the period of time when your body is saying, "Hold tight; changes are afoot!"

Hormonal Changes: The Ringleaders of the Circus

Hormones are those little chemicals darting around in your blood-stream that make you, well, you. But during perimenopause, they're also the ones stirring the pot. Oestrogen and progesterone levels fluctuate, leading to a host of changes in your body. It's a bit like a seesaw that can't quite find its balance. One moment you're up, and the next, you're not so up. You're basically hosting a hormonal soirée, and not everyone on the guest list plays nicely together.

A Plethora of Symptoms: From A to Z

When it comes to symptoms, perimenopause has a buffet to offer. Hot flushes? Check. Sleep disruptions? Oh yes. Mood swings? Welcome to the club. There are also irregular periods, weight gain, fatigue, and decreased libido to name but a few. According to a study in the *Journal of Women's Health*, up to 87% of women experience hot flushes during this period. That's almost as high as the percentage of us who love a good cup of tea on a chilly day (100%, in case you were wondering). So, you're most certainly not alone, even when it feels like your body is pulling pranks on you.

Inclusivity Matters: Non-Binary and Trans Men

Non-binary individuals and trans men who have not had surgery or hormonal treatments affecting their ovaries may also experience this transitional phase too. Although research is still a bit limited in this area, it's crucial to recognise that perimenopause is an inclusive affair. As always, consult healthcare professionals for advice tailored to your needs.

Premature Ovarian Insufficiency (POI)

Sometimes, life throws a curveball, or in this case, POI. Premature ovarian insufficiency is a condition where the ovaries lose their normal function before the age of 40. It's not the same as perimenopause, although some symptoms might overlap. Unlike perimenopause, POI can make it more difficult for women to conceive and may necessitate hormone replacement therapy at a younger age. According to the NHS, about one in a hundred women experience POI.

Knowledge is Power

Understanding perimenopause isn't just about coming to terms with biological changes; it's about embracing a new chapter in your life. Sure, it might be a bit of a tumultuous chapter, but think of all the wisdom that comes with it. As Eleanor Roosevelt said,

"With the new day comes new strength and new thoughts."

So, grab each new day of your perimenopausal journey with both hands, and remember, you've got the strength and wisdom to navigate through this phase like the amazing woman you are. Take the information in this book as your shield and sword, as you transition into a perimenopause warrior. Here's to conquering perimenopause, one hot flush at a time!

CHAPTER 3

THE HORMONAL HOKEY COKEY

What's really going on inside you?

In the grand tapestry of life, the story woven by hormones is one of grace, balance and continual renewal. Each hormone weaves its thread into this complex and exquisite design, embodying distinct roles yet harmoniously collaborating to create the vibrant, evolving portrait of a woman's life. As we step into the golden chapter of perimenopause, it often feels like this hormonal dance is more like the hokey cokey – trying to get everyone together to hold hands, but some rushing in whilst others feel like they're rushing out – and lots of shaking of different body parts too!

Oestrogen – The Fountain of Vitality

Oestrogen is one of the main hormones responsible for regulating the menstrual cycle and maintaining pregnancy, among other things. When oestrogen levels are steady, all is generally well in the kingdom of reproductive health. However, during perimenopause, the production of this crucial hormone starts to fluctuate before eventually declining. This hormonal shift is primarily due to the ovaries winding down their reproductive capabilities.

In the years leading up to menopause, the number of ovarian follicles – a combination of eggs and the cells surrounding them decreases. With fewer follicles, there's less oestrogen production. In essence, your ovaries are taking their last bow and slowly exiting the reproductive stage. Some studies indicate a decrease in oestrogen levels by up to 35% during this period. The term 'decline' may sound a bit negative, but it's a completely natural part of the ageing process. It's like your body's way of saying, "I've been working hard for decades; it's time to shift gears."

The variance in oestrogen levels isn't just a steady decline; it can also be quite erratic, especially in the early stages of perimenopause. You may experience periods of relatively high oestrogen, sometimes described as 'oestrogen surges,' followed by abrupt drops. These fluctuations can make symptoms feel like a roller coaster of physiological and emotional changes. You might find yourself experiencing hot flushes one moment and chills the next. You may notice changes in your menstrual cycle – sometimes it's shorter, sometimes longer, and sometimes it takes a holiday without notifying you!

This ebb and flow of oestrogen also have more long-term effects on your body. For instance, the decrease in oestrogen levels can contribute to bone density loss, making bones more susceptible to fractures. It's not just the bones; lower oestrogen affects the cardiovascular system too. Changes in cholesterol levels, specifically an increase in LDL (the 'bad' cholesterol) and a decrease in HDL (the 'good' cholesterol), can be influenced by lower oestrogen, thereby affecting heart health. While the decline in oestrogen might seem overwhelming, understanding its effects can empower you to take proactive measures for your well-being which I will discuss in later chapters.

Progesterone – One of the Feel-Good Hormones

Often playing second fiddle to its more talked-about counterpart, oestrogen, progesterone has its own crucial roles in the body. This hormone is vital for regulating the menstrual cycle and is particularly important in the second half of the cycle, post-ovulation, preparing the uterine lining for a potential pregnancy.

In the grand symphony of perimenopause, progesterone also sees a decline, and understanding its diminishing levels can be just as crucial. Unlike oestrogen, which can have erratic levels in early perimenopause, progesterone's decline is generally more straightforward. Why? Well, as we age, the frequency of ovulation decreases. Each time an ovary releases an egg, the body produces progesterone; hence fewer ovulation events mean less progesterone production. In essence, when ovulation becomes less frequent, the production of progesterone takes a nosedive as well.

The decline in progesterone can create an imbalance between it and oestrogen. This imbalance can manifest itself in several ways. For instance, you may notice changes in your menstrual cycles, which may become heavier and more prolonged. Progesterone's role in stabilising the lining of the uterus means that lower levels can lead to more intense periods. In some studies, it's been shown that heavier menstrual cycles during perimenopause are linked with this decline in progesterone.

Another intriguing impact of progesterone's decline is mood swings and sleep disturbances. Progesterone has a calming effect and helps regulate sleep patterns. Lower levels can result in disrupted sleep and increased anxiety for some people. It's as if your internal metronome that usually keeps things ticking along smoothly has decided to take some unexpected breaks.

Managing the decline in progesterone involves a multi-faceted approach. Hormone replacement therapy (HRT) often includes both oestrogen and progesterone, especially for women who still have their uterus, to ensure a balanced hormonal environment. Lifestyle interventions, like regular exercise and stress-management techniques such as mindfulness and meditation, can also offer symptomatic relief. Again, I'll talk about this in later chapters in more detail.

Testosterone is Not Just for Men

This hormone is often associated with men – for me, I always think of big bulky guys in the gym – but it's actually a vital player in women's health as well. It's like the unsung hero of the hormonal trio, including oestrogen and progesterone, that keeps our bodies ticking along smoothly. While testosterone is known for its role in libido, it also contributes to muscle mass, bone density, and even our mood.

As with oestrogen and progesterone, testosterone levels also experience a decline during perimenopause. But it's worth noting that the decline in testosterone actually begins earlier, often starting in a woman's late 20s or early 30s. By the time you reach perimenopause, you might already have lower levels of testosterone compared to your younger years. However, the perimenopausal years often see an accelerated decrease. Some studies indicate that women could experience a drop in testosterone levels by up to 25% during this period.

Why does testosterone decline? One reason is that the ovaries, which produce a significant portion of testosterone, become less active in producing this hormone as we age. Also, increased levels of sex hormone-binding globulin (SHBG) during perimenopause can bind to testosterone, making less of it available for use by the body.

The decline in testosterone can have an array of effects. You may notice a drop in your libido, which is one of the more well-documented symptoms associated with reduced testosterone. However, the impact goes beyond the bedroom. Lower levels of testosterone are linked with decreased muscle mass and a reduction in overall energy levels. Remember that pep in your step? Lower testosterone might have carted some of it away.

It's not just the physical aspect; the psychological impact can be significant too. A reduction in testosterone levels has been associated with brain fog, mood swings, and even increased symptoms of anxiety or depression in some cases. While testosterone is not the sole influencer of our emotional well-being, its decline can contribute to the mood variations that some women experience during perimenopause.

Like with the other hormonal declines, the lower levels of testosterone can be managed. Some women turn to hormone replacement therapy (HRT) that includes testosterone, although this approach is still a topic of ongoing research and discussion and not (yet) available on the NHS. Non-hormonal options include lifestyle changes such as regular exercise, particularly strength training, to boost muscle mass and improve bone density. Adequate sleep and stress management can also support better hormonal balance, including stabilising testosterone levels.

The Duet of FSH and LH

Now, let's talk about two other essential players in the perimenopausal ensemble: follicle stimulating hormone (FSH) and luteinising hormone (LH). These hormones might not be the headline acts like oestrogen and progesterone, but they're the conductors that keep the hormonal orchestra in tune. They originate from the pituitary gland and are vital in controlling the menstrual cycle. But when perimenopause comes knocking, their levels start to dance to a different tune.

In a curious twist, FSH levels actually tend to rise during perimenopause. You might wonder, "Wait a minute, isn't everything supposed to be declining?" Well, FSH levels increase because the hormone is working overtime to encourage the ovaries to produce a viable egg. It's as if FSH is shaking the proverbial tree harder and harder each month to see what falls out. As the ovaries become less responsive due to ageing, more FSH is produced in an attempt to stimulate the ovaries into action. Some women could see FSH levels rise considerably, sometimes even doubling, during perimenopause.

LH levels, on the other hand, can also rise but not as dramatically as FSH. LH is responsible for triggering ovulation and stimulating the corpus luteum (the remains of the ovarian follicle) to produce progesterone. With less frequent ovulation during perimenopause, you'd think LH might decline. However, like FSH, LH levels often increase as the body attempts to prompt the ovaries to keep up their end of the reproductive bargain.

These hormonal fluctuations have real-world implications for your symptoms and experiences during perimenopause. For instance, a spike in FSH levels could be responsible for those shorter menstrual cycles at the beginning of perimenopause. It's like FSH saying, "We're in a hurry, let's move things along!" Moreover, higher levels of FSH and LH can contribute to menstrual irregularities, which many women experience during this transitional phase.

From a diagnostic standpoint, physicians often measure FSH levels to determine if a woman is entering perimenopause or menopause, although it's not always a definitive indicator due to its fluctuating nature. Some studies have shown that FSH levels can swing widely in short periods, making a single measurement less meaningful, and why testing in perimenopause can be unreliable. See chapter5 on testing.

So, while perimenopause may feel like a hormonal roller coaster (with more ups and downs than you may care for), understanding the roles of FSH and LH provides a valuable roadmap for what's going on inside your body. Various strategies that we'll look at, from hormone replacement therapy to lifestyle adjustments, can help you deal with these hormonal changes more effectively.

Cortisol

Moving on to yet another hormone that gets swept into the perimenopausal tide: cortisol. Often termed the 'stress hormone,' cortisol is released by the adrenal glands and plays an essential role in various bodily functions such as metabolism, immune response, and, yes, stress management. Unlike FSH and LH, cortisol doesn't directly regulate reproductive functions, but it does have a profound influence on how we experience perimenopause.

During perimenopause, the relationship between cortisol and other hormones becomes a bit like a seesaw. While cortisol levels don't necessarily decline as a part of the perimenopausal process, imbalances in other hormones can affect how cortisol functions or is perceived in the body. For example, the irregular levels of oestrogen can make the body more sensitive to cortisol, amplifying feelings of stress and anxiety. It's a bit like turning up the volume on your emotional responses; suddenly, small irritations can feel like monumental challenges.

Interestingly, elevated cortisol levels can have a knock-on effect on other hormones. Elevated cortisol can inhibit the release of luteinising hormone (LH), which, as we know, plays a crucial role in ovulation and reproductive health. So, even though cortisol doesn't decline in a way that oestrogen, progesterone, and testosterone do, its levels can still be impacted by the hormonal fluctuations that are par for the course in perimenopause.

Symptoms? Oh, there are symptoms. Chronic stress, exacerbated by higher cortisol sensitivity, can result in weight gain, particularly around the abdomen. Stress-induced eating, anyone? Furthermore, elevated cortisol levels can disrupt sleep patterns, leading to sleep deprivation. This can create a vicious cycle, as lack of sleep can also elevate cortisol levels, making you feel even more stressed. It's like your body's own version of a 'catch 22.'

The repercussions don't stop there. High levels of cortisol can also affect bone density, muscle mass, and even cognitive functions like memory and concentration. In essence, while cortisol may not decline during perimenopause, its impact can be more pronounced due to the hormonal cocktail of this life stage.

Managing cortisol levels during perimenopause often involves stress-reducing techniques. Exercise is a proven method for reducing cortisol levels, with some studies suggesting that even moderate exercise can result in a 20-30% reduction in the stress hormone. Mindfulness practices, adequate sleep, and a balanced diet can also contribute to stabilising cortisol levels.

So, although cortisol might not be declining in the same way as our other hormonal characters, its role in the perimenopausal story is far from a cameo. Understanding its interactions with other hormones and its heightened impact during this phase can arm you with the information you need to navigate perimenopause with grace, resilience, and, ideally, a lot less stress.

See chapter 6 on stress.

The Balance

As we close this enlightening journey through the hormonal landscape of perimenopause, let's take a moment to discuss the harmony – or sometimes discord – that exists between these different hormones. It's less a solo performance and more an intricate ballet, with each hormone playing its unique part in creating the dance that is perimenopause.

The balance between oestrogen, progesterone, testosterone, cortisol, FSH, and LH is delicately orchestrated, almost like a well-conducted symphony. During perimenopause, however, it's as if someone switched the sheet music, creating fluctuations and imbalances that your body needs to learn to adapt to.

This dynamic equilibrium of hormones may seem overwhelming, but it's your body's natural way of transitioning to a new phase of life. Despite the challenges, it's worth remembering that for many, life post-menopause is met with a newfound sense of freedom and relief from many of the symptoms experienced during perimenopause.

So, as we reach the end of this hormonal voyage, the message is one of empowerment. Yes, perimenopause is a complex and often challenging time, but it's also a transition that nearly half the population goes through. You're far from alone on this journey. With the right support and information, this chapter of your life can be a transformative and positive experience.

In the words of Maya Angelou,

"We delight in the beauty of the butterfly,

but rarely admit the changes it has gone through to achieve that beauty."

Here's to embracing the changes of perimenopause and emerging as your most empowered, vibrant self.

CHAPTER 4

Perimenopause Symptoms

The who's who

Welcome to the chapter that could very well be considered the 'Who's Who' of perimenopausal symptoms. Now, before you even glance at the list of 111 symptoms and consider packing your bags for a one-way trip to a secluded island, let's take a deep breath together. While it's true that perimenopause can bring about a myriad of changes – some welcomed, others not so much – it's important to remember that this phase is as much a rite of passage as it is a hormonal roller coaster.

Think of this chapter as your comprehensive guide, your A to Z – or shall we say, your hot flushes to sleep disturbances – of what you might encounter during this fascinating life stage. But here's the silver lining: Not every woman will experience every symptom. In fact, you might go through perimenopause with just a handful of these symptoms making guest appearances.

It's as Forrest Gump so eloquently put it: "Life is like a box of chocolates; you never know what you're going to get." In the context of perimenopause, each symptom is like a different chocolate in the assortment. Some might be to your liking, or at least manageable, while others may have you wondering who on earth thought that particular filling was a good idea. But remember, even if you encounter a less-than-pleasant strawberry cream – my personal 'ick' – that one flavour (symptom) doesn't have to define the whole box.

While the list is extensive, the purpose is not to overwhelm you but to empower you. Fore-warned is forearmed, as they say. With this detailed roadmap, you'll be better equipped to recognise and understand what's happening to your body, thereby making it easier to seek the appropriate remedies or medical advice.

Another point to consider is that each symptom is a clue, a signal from your body asking for attention. Whether it's introducing dietary changes, ramping up your exercise routine, or perhaps trying hormone replacement therapy, there are a myriad of ways to manage these symptoms. You don't have to grit your teeth and bear it; you have options, lots of them.

In the wise words of Eleanor Roosevelt,

"Women are like teabags. We don't know our true strength until we are in hot water."

While the hot water of perimenopause might come with mood swings and memory lapses, it's also an opportunity to tap into your reservoirs of resilience and ingenuity.

So, as you read through this comprehensive list of symptoms, take it one step at a time. Remember, knowledge is power. By understanding what's in store, you'll be better prepared to navigate the labyrinth that is perimenopause, coming out the other side not just unscathed but triumphantly empowered.

I will also be going into detail, later in this book, about what causes the different symptoms, what you can do to help, and when you should consult your healthcare provider

Difficulty Concentrating and Memory Lapse

1. **Difficulty concentrating**: Ever find yourself reading the same line three times? A common symptom that can be quite frustrating.

2. **Memory lapse**: Momentary forgetfulness, like forgetting where you placed your keys or forgetting names.

3. **Brain fog**: A feeling of mental cloudiness, making it hard to think clearly.

4. **Difficulty finding words**: When words are on the tip of your tongue but refuse to make an appearance.

5. **Impaired judgment**: Decision-making can become more challenging during this phase.

6. **Increased clumsiness**: Suddenly bumping into furniture? It's not just you.

Mental Health and Mindset

7. **Anxiety**: Elevated worry or stress that can be debilitating at times.

8. **Depression**: Persistent low mood that goes beyond mere sadness.

9. **Feeling dead inside**: Emotional numbness.

10. **Disconnection from loved ones/partner**: A sense of emotional distance from those around you.

11. **Irritability**: Feeling easily annoyed or angered.

12. **Panic attacks/disorder**: Sudden episodes of intense fear.

13. **Decreased libido**: Lowered interest in sexual activities.

14. **Muscle tension**: Stiffness or tightness in the muscles, often due to stress.

15. **Fatigue**: Persistent tiredness that doesn't seem to go away.

16. **Disrupted sleep**: Difficulty maintaining a consistent sleep schedule.

17. **Insomnia**: Persistent difficulty falling or staying asleep.

18. **Mood swings**: Rapid changes in mood, often for no discernible reason.

19. **Crying spells**: Sudden episodes of crying without a clear cause.

20. **Feeling overwhelmed**: A sense of not being able to cope with day-to-day tasks.

21. **Increased vulnerability to stress**: Stressors have a greater impact than they used to.

22. **Decreased self-esteem**: Feeling less confident about oneself.

23. **Feeling disconnected from others**: A sense of isolation or detachment.

24. **Loss of interest in previously enjoyed activities**: Things that once brought joy no longer do.

25. **Decreased motivation**: Reduced drive to achieve goals.

Weight Gain, Bloating, and Changes in Body Composition

26. **Weight gain**: Unexplained increase in body weight.

27. **Bloating**: Swelling or puffiness in the abdominal area.

28. **Gas**: Excessive flatulence.

29. **Changes in body composition**: Shifting of fat distribution, often towards the abdominal area.

Digestive and Stomach Problems, and Diarrhoea [and metabolism]

30. **Digestive problems**: Issues like indigestion or heartburn.

31. **Diarrhoea**: Frequent, loose bowel movements.

32. **Abdominal pain**: Pain or discomfort in the stomach area.

33. **Dry mouth**: A parched feeling that's hard to shake off.

34. **Gum problems**: Issues like gingivitis or increased sensitivity.

35. **Food cravings**: A sudden, intense desire for specific foods.

36. **Changes in appetite**: Either a loss of appetite or excessive hunger.

37. **Nausea**: Persistent or frequent feelings of queasiness.

38. **Changes in blood sugar levels**: Fluctuating levels of glucose in the blood.

39. **Increased risk of diabetes**: A heightened chance of developing type 2 diabetes.

40. **Burning tongue**: A scalding sensation in the tongue without an apparent reason.

41. **Difficulty swallowing**: Challenges in moving food from mouth to stomach.

42. **Increased sensitivity to alcohol or caffeine**: Even small amounts can have a strong effect.

Urinary Problems, Frequent Urination, and Stress Incontinence

43. **Stress incontinence**: Involuntary leaking of urine when you cough, laugh, or sneeze.

44. **Urinary problems**: Issues like frequent urges or pain during urination.

45. **Urinary tract infections**: Infections affecting any part of the urinary system.

46. **Frequent urination**: Needing to go more often than usual.

47. **Frequent urination at night**: Multiple trips to the loo disrupting your sleep.

Vaginal Dryness and Atrophy

48. **Vaginal dryness**: Reduced moisture leading to discomfort.

49. **Vaginal atrophy**: Thinning and inflammation of the vaginal walls.

Headaches/Migraines

50. **Headaches**: Persistent or frequent headaches, often tension related.

51. **Migraines**: Severe headaches often accompanied by nausea and light sensitivity.

Heart Palpitations and Irregular Heartbeat

52. **Irregular heartbeat**: Heart skipping beats or beating too fast/slow.

53. **Heart palpitations**: Feeling like your heart is pounding, fluttering, or beating irregularly.

54. **Increased blood pressure**: Consistently high readings.

55. **Increased risk of cardiovascular disease**: Elevated chance of heart-related issues.

Menstrual Cycle Changes

56. **Longer menstrual cycles**: Periods spaced further apart.

57. **Irregular periods**: Unpredictable menstrual cycles.

58. **Changes in menstrual flow**: Either too heavy or too light.

59. **Heavy periods**: Excessive bleeding.

60. **Light periods**: Very minimal bleeding.

61. **Shorter menstrual cycles**: Periods coming more frequently.

62. **Spotting between periods**: Light bleeding outside of regular menstrual cycles.

63. **Changes in menstrual cycle length**: Variability in the duration between periods.

64. **Increased menstrual cramps**: More severe or frequent pain.

65. **PMS-like symptoms**: Experiencing premenstrual symptoms more intensely.

66. **Worsening of premenstrual syndrome (PMS)**: Increased severity of PMS symptoms.

Skin and Nails

67. **Formication**: Sensation of insects crawling on your skin.

68. **Dry skin**: Less natural oil production leading to dryness.

69. **Itchy skin**: Persistent or frequent itching.

70. **Itchy ears**: Unexplained itchiness in the ear canal.

71. **Acne**: Increased outbreaks.

72. **Brittle nails**: Nails become fragile and easily breakable.

73. **Body odour changes**: Altered scent, not always for the better!

74. **Increased tendency to bruise**: Bruises appear more easily.

75. **Itchy scalp**: Persistent scalp itchiness.

76. **Facial flushing**: Redness or a warm feeling in the face.

77. **Loss of elasticity in the skin**: Skin becoming less supple.

78. **Skin discolouration**: Dark spots or uneven skin tone.

Hair Changes – Thinning Hair, Hair Loss, and Brittle Hair

79. **Thinning hair**: Reduced hair density.

80. **More facial hair**: Increased hair growth on the face.

81. **Hair loss**: More hair falling out than usual.

82. **Brittle hair**: Hair breaking easily.

Changes in Sensation

83. **Dizzy spells**: Sudden, unexplained feelings of dizziness.

84. **Tinnitus**: Ringing in the ears.

85. **Phantom smells**: Detecting smells that aren't actually there.

86. **Vertigo**: Sensation of spinning or dizziness when still.

87. **Restless legs syndrome**: An irresistible urge to move your legs.

88. **Changes in vision**: Like blurriness or increased sensitivity to light.

89. **Sensitivity to noise**: Sounds seem louder or more irritating.

90. **Changes in sense of taste**: Foods may taste differently.

91. **Restlessness**: Feeling of constant unease or nervousness.

92. **Electric shock-like sensations in the head**: Feeling of electrical surges in the head.

93. **Sensation of electric shocks**: Jolts of electricity running through the body.

94. **Tingling extremities**: Numbness or tingling in hands and feet.

95. **Loss of balance**: Feeling unsteady on your feet.

Vasomotor Symptoms

96. **Hot flushes**: Sudden intense heat sensations.

97. **Cold flashes**: Opposite of hot flushes, sudden chills.

98. **Changes in body temperature regulation**: Overheating or feeling unusually cold.

99. **Night sweats**: Waking up soaked in sweat.

Muscle, Joints, and Bones

100. **Joint pain**: Aching or stiffness in joints.

101. **Frozen shoulder**: Pain and stiffness in the shoulder joint.

102. **Osteoporosis**: Weakening of bones, making them fragile.

103. **Muscle aches**: Persistent muscle pain.

Physiological Changes [otherwise unclassified]

104. **Increased susceptibility to infections**: Getting sick more often than usual.

105. **Breast soreness/tenderness**: Unexplained pain in the breast area.

106. **Shortness of breath**: Difficulty in breathing during activities that were once easy.

107. **Chest pain**: Unexplained pain or tightness in the chest.

108. **Allergies or sensitivities**: New or heightened reactions to substances.

109. **Dry eyes**: Eyes feeling itchy or sandy.

110. **Sudden high cholesterol (also called dyslipidaemia)**: Unexplained increase in cholesterol levels.

111. **Breast swelling**: Unexplained increase in breast size.

I know, it's a long list, but remember not every woman will experience all of these symptoms. Some might only encounter a few, and the intensity can vary from person to person. Think of it like a buffet, where you get to pick what you want to deal with. And even if you do encounter a more challenging symptom, treatments and strategies are available to help you manage. Stay encouraged and informed – you're not alone in this journey!

If you would like a checklist of these symptoms that you could use for yourself, or show to your medical professional to discuss possible treatment plans, you can find them in *The UncompliKated Perimenopause Journal* or pop to www.myperimenopausesymptoms.com to download a copy for free.

CHAPTER 5

The Perimeno-pause Puzzle

To test or not to test, that is the question

Introduction: The British Dilemma

We British have a certain love for queues and order. We like our tea hot, our humour dry, and our medical diagnoses clear-cut. But when it comes to perimenopause, things can get a bit, well, foggy. Many GPs are still under the impression that they need to 'test' for perimenopause to 'treat' it with hormone replacement therapy (HRT). But is that really the case? I beg to differ.

The Unreliable Blood Test: A Tale of Two Hormones

Navigating the perimenopausal waters is challenging enough without being presented with another curveball: the unreliable blood test. Imagine going for a blood test expecting to unlock the mysteries of your hormonal fluctuations, only to find out the results are as reliable as a magic 8-ball. Yet that's the predicament many women find themselves in when trying to diagnose perimenopause through blood tests measuring FSH (follicle stimulating hormone) and LH (luteinising hormone).

According to medical literature, these hormone levels can fluctuate so wildly that using them as a diagnostic tool for women over 45 is considered unreliable. One study even suggests that blood tests miss the diagnosis up to 30% of the time for perimenopausal women. That's not exactly a glowing endorsement for a test that's supposed to help clarify things. It's like trying to predict the outcome of a football match by only watching the first ten minutes – entertaining, but not very insightful.

It's not all doom and gloom, however. Guidelines from the National Institute for Health and Care Excellence (NICE) in the UK suggest that blood tests aren't the be-all-and-end-all- for perimenopausal diagnosis (see more on this below). Instead, healthcare providers are advised to look at the full picture, including a thorough review of symptoms, menstrual history, and other relevant health factors. So, if your GP starts brandishing a syringe and talking blood tests, it might be more helpful to discuss the broader landscape of your symptoms instead.

Self-Help Strategies

Keep a Symptoms Diary: Documenting your symptoms can provide a clearer picture than fluctuating hormones ever could. It might just be your best tool in proactive healthcare at this stage. You can find this in the accompanying journal to this book (*The UncompliKated Perimenopause Journal*).

Or you could download a copy by going to www.myperimenopuasesymptoms.com

Consult Multiple Sources: Don't be shy to get a second or even third opinion. Sometimes it takes a village to diagnose a hormonal shift.

Look for Patterns: If you're tracking symptoms and still getting blood tests, look for correlations. Even if the hormones themselves are unreliable, trends can offer insights.

Stay Informed: Familiarise yourself with NICE guidelines or other reputable sources. When it comes to your health, knowledge really is power.

Alternative Diagnostic Methods: Consider other diagnostic methods like saliva tests or basal body temperature tracking, although these are not without their own limitations.

Communication: Always maintain open communication with your healthcare provider. Their experience combined with your detailed symptoms diary can form a powerful diagnostic team.

So, while diagnosing perimenopause might sometimes feel like cracking the Da Vinci Code, remember that you're not just a hormone level to be measured – you're a whole, complicated, wonderful human being experiencing a normal phase of life. With the right approach and information, you can navigate this stage with grit and grace.

The NICE Guidelines: The Voice of Reason

The National Institute for Health and Care Excellence (NICE) has guidelines that are, well, rather nice. If you're over 45 and you've turned into a human thermostat experiencing hot flushes and night sweats, along with menstrual irregularities, you can give the needle a skip.

According to NICE, you can head straight to discussing treatment options based on your symptoms. This is great news, as it places the emphasis on the lived experience of women going through perimenopause rather than arbitrary hormone levels. In fact, a review of NICE's 2015 guidelines on the diagnosis and management of menopause states that blood tests are not necessary for women aged 45 or over who have menopausal symptoms. That's a weight off, especially for anyone with a phobia of needles, or who just wants to get on with managing symptoms.

So, if you're headed to a healthcare appointment, preparation is key. Use my free checklist and tracker at www.myperimenopausesymptoms.com, or see the accompanying journal to this book if you prefer a hardcopy, to list down your symptoms. This is like bringing a detailed roadmap to your consultation – super helpful for you and a lifesaver for your healthcare provider. According to feedback from many women who've used my checklist/tracker, this approach can be transformative. When it comes to discussing your symptoms with your healthcare provider, there's nothing quite like showing up armed with a well-documented arsenal of what you're going through. Suddenly, you're not just saying you're experiencing hot flushes; you can specify their frequency, triggers, and impact on your life.

Self-Help Strategies

Preparation is Half the Battle: Before your appointment, gather all your symptoms together, preferably in a checklist or tracker. It doesn't only have to be physical symptoms; emotional and psychological ones count too.

Speak the Language: Familiarise yourself with the NICE guidelines. This ensures you and your healthcare provider are literally on the same page. I've included a glossary of terms at the back of this book if there are any terms you're not yet familiar with.

Open Dialogue: Don't hesitate to ask questions. You're not at a quiz show, but knowledge is indeed power here. The more you understand about your condition and the guidelines, the more empowered you'll be.

Involve Your Healthcare Provider: Make sure to show them your checklist and tracker. This opens up the floor for a more nuanced discussion on treatment options.

Advocate for Yourself: If your healthcare provider suggests a blood test despite you fitting the NICE criteria, gently remind them of the guidelines. Sometimes healthcare providers need refreshers too!

Know Your Treatment Options: Once diagnosed, there's a plethora of treatment routes to explore – HRT, non-hormonal medications, lifestyle changes, and so on. Your checklist can serve as a guide here as well, helping to pinpoint which treatments might be most effective for your particular set of symptoms. See chapters 24-29 for healing levels.

So, there you have it. NICE guidelines are your back-pocket tool for navigating the perimenopausal labyrinth. Armed with your symptom's tracker, you're not just throwing darts in the dark; you're engaging in an informed discussion about your health. And that's pretty much the adult version of winning a gold star sticker, if you ask me.

The Under-45 Conundrum: A Different Ball Game

If you are in the under-45 bracket – the age group where you're not quite sure if your symptoms are a midlife preamble or you just had too much spicy food last night – you're caught between a rock and a hot flash, so to speak. It's a tricky one, no doubt.

Firstly, being under 45 puts you in a special category because, generally, perimenopausal symptoms are less expected (theoretically, you can still have them). At this age, your GP might raise an eyebrow and even consider other possibilities like premature ovarian insufficiency (POI) – see more on this below, which affects about 1 in 100 women under 40 according to the NHS. That's a small but significant number, so it's on the radar.

But, my lovely, I really want you to know that it can genuinely be the perimenopause – even if you're in your late 30s or early 40s. Track your symptoms and get really well informed (this book is a great resource for that) because the more well-versed you are, the more gravity you lend to your discussions with your doctor. Don't give up, and reach out to me, and the other wonderful women, in my Facebook group if you need support (Perimenopause with Kate Grosvenor).

Self-Help Strategies

Be Proactive, Not Reactive: Make a comprehensive list of your symptoms. It's a bit like writing your CV, but instead of job experiences, you're listing all the weird things happening to your body. The more thorough you are, the easier it'll be for your healthcare provider to see the bigger picture.

Be Ready for Tests: Your GP may recommend hormone tests to rule out POI or other conditions, especially if you're under 40. According to guidelines by the American College of Obstetricians and Gynaecologists (ACOG), women under 40 experiencing perimenopausal symptoms should be evaluated for causes like POI.

A Second Opinion Never Hurts: If your GP is adamant about tests, but you feel like your symptoms are textbook perimenopause, don't be shy about seeking a second opinion. Sometimes two heads (or two doctors) are better than one.

Consider HRT: Some doctors may feel confident prescribing hormone replacement therapy (HRT) even without blood tests if your symptoms strongly suggest perimenopause. About 10% of women experience early menopause before the age of 45, and HRT can be particularly beneficial for this group, according to the British Menopause Society. (See more on HRT later in this book).

Alternative Therapies: Don't overlook lifestyle changes and natural remedies. A balanced diet, regular exercise, and stress management techniques can go a long way in easing perimenopausal symptoms.

Do Your Research: Be familiar with the guidelines relevant to your age group, whether it's NICE or ACOG. The more educated you are, the more empowered you'll be in your healthcare journey. After all, knowledge is power. But here, it could also mean the difference between endless tests and effective treatment.

Document, Document, Document: Keep track of your symptoms and any treatments you've tried. A well-documented case makes it easier for your healthcare provider to offer you the best care possible.

So, if you're under 45 and experiencing what feels like perimenopausal symptoms, it's not the end of the world; it's just a more complicated chapter of the book. But remember, this is a phase of life, and just like your teenage years, it too shall pass. By being proactive and well-informed, you're setting yourself up for the best possible outcomes.

The Additional Tests: The American Way

Across the pond in the USA, doctors often go a step further. They might conduct additional tests to rule out other issues related to thyroid function, blood sugar, liver function, and vitamin levels like D, B12, and iron. It's like the medical version of the American 'more is more' philosophy. But remember, the NICE guidelines clearly state that treatment should be based on symptoms, not blood test results.

The Final Verdict: Listen to Your Body

The NICE guidelines are straightforward: people should be treated with HRT based on their symptoms, not blood test results. So, if you're sitting in your GP's office, feeling like you're having your own private summer in the middle of a British winter, trust your body. It's telling you something important.

Further Reading and Resources

For those who want to delve deeper into the guidelines and what they mean for you, if you pop 'NICE guidelines' into your search engine, you'll go straight to the information. I've listed the website in 'Helpful Resources' at the end of this book.

So, my darling, the next time you find yourself in your doctor's office debating whether or not to get that blood test, remember this chapter. Trust your symptoms, know the guidelines, and maybe, just maybe, you'll find that navigating the perimenopause maze isn't as complicated as it seems.

CHAPTER 6

From Stress Fest to Zen Zone

Your guide to keeping calm in the perimenopause chaos

As we discussed, this period in your life can be full of stories of growth, transformation, and newfound wisdom. However, this is also intertwined with a myriad of stressors that sometimes overshadow the more positive journey of self-discovery and empowerment.

At this pivotal juncture, women stand at the crossroads of multiple life phases, often juggling the nurturing demands of family, the fulfilling yet sometimes taxing endeavours of career growth, and perhaps, whispering goodbyes to the children leaving home. It's a time when our roles may shift, and these shifts can bring forth a cascade of responsibilities and expectations, sometimes harmonious, yet at times overwhelming and seem to almost bury us with its intensity.

Furthermore, during this transformative period, women find ourselves amidst a whirlpool of conflicting roles– a nurturing mother, a devoted partner, a blossoming individual – there are so many, and the juggling act needed sometimes becomes fast-paced and complex with elements of stress thrown into the narrative of our lives.

The physical narrative also chimes in, adding to it all. The hormonal turmoil, that has played seamlessly in the background for years, now comes to the forefront, sometimes missing a beat, sometimes changing the tempo abruptly. These fluctuating hormones can sometimes manifest as physical discomforts, erratic sleep patterns, and shifting moods, requiring a deft touch and grace to navigate seamlessly.

Yet amidst this disarray lies an opportunity, a golden moment to pause, to tune into one's own rhythmic heartbeat. It's a call to embrace the harmony within, to curate a new chapter that resonates with tranquillity and balance.

Therefore, as we delve deeper into this chapter of stress and perimenopause, and the complex relationship between the two, it is important to realise that a nurturing idea of self, a prioritising of self-care, and an attitude of doing 'whatever it takes' is the secret recipe to smoothing over the troubled times.

The Cortisol-Progesterone Battle

I mentioned cortisol in the earlier chapter earlier on hormones, but we need to discuss it in more detail.

Cortisol and progesterone share a complex relationship. In the midst of stressful times, the body may prioritise the production of cortisol, somewhat hijacking the resources needed to produce progesterone, a vital hormone that aids in regulating the menstrual cycle and fostering a sense of calmness. This phenomenon is popularly known as the 'progesterone steal'.

In perimenopause, the 'progesterone steal' plays a critical role. During periods of stress, our bodies tend to prioritise the production of cortisol, a hormone vital for responding to stress, quite zealously. This process, unfortunately, diverts the precursors that would typically be used to create progesterone, leading to a dip in its production. This shift can sometimes result in heightened feelings of anxiety, mood swings, and disruptions in menstrual cycles, as the harmonious balance gets somewhat skewed.

Self-Help Strategies

Understanding the dynamics of the progesterone steal allows you to take proactive steps in managing stress levels thereby nurturing the delicate balance between cortisol and progesterone.

Grounding Activities: Consider activities that ground you, like meditation or a walk in the park, as ways to foster balance and harmony. Or maybe an activity like swimming – it's low-impact and offers not only a full-body workout, but it helps you to feel balanced too.

Nurturing & Soothing: To help foster a harmonious balance between cortisol and progesterone, focus on nurturing and self-soothing activities that evoke peace and serenity, such as a warm bubble bath infused with lavender oil or a gentle walk amidst nature.

Mindfulness and Relaxation: This will sincerely bring more balance. Even just 10 minutes of meditation a day can help reduce cortisol and improve your mental state too. Progressive muscle relaxation – which is like a body scan that involves tensing and relaxing muscles from the toes upwards – promoted both physical and mental relaxation.

Creative Outlets: Ideas such as journaling, just writing down your thoughts, can be incredibly therapeutic. Art and craft activities, such as painting or knitting, can be meditative too and lower stress. Whereas music, either listening to or playing, can elevate your moods also lowering cortisol levels.

The Story of Serotonin

Serotonin – our 'feel-good' neurotransmitter – affects our mood, happiness, and sleep. The fluctuations in hormone levels during perimenopause can affect serotonin levels , occasionally leading to dips in mood and increased anxiety. Fortunately, with a nurturing approach toward diet and lifestyle, we can guide serotonin to optimal levels again.

A big help here is to cultivate a serotonin-nourishing garden in your daily diet. Include foods rich in tryptophan, such as turkey, bananas, pineapples, and eggs, accompanied by a daily dose of sunshine and laughter, nurturing serotonin's graceful waltz in your body.

When you are traversing through the perimenopausal phase, crafting resilience is of the utmost importance. Incorporating nurturing practices such as yoga and meditation can guide the erratic energies of stress into a gentle flow, fostering a tranquil dance of serenity and poise.

According to a study published in the Journal of Women's Health, incorporating a regimen of yoga significantly helped women mitigate the symptoms of perimenopause, fostering a space of tranquillity and balance within.

Before perimenopause started for me, I was always into a tad, let's say, energetic sports. It was all about hockey, tennis, or boxing. Anything that involved smacking a ball or punching a bag was my 'thing'. It helped me to let off steam. However, what I most need now is peace and quiet, to breathe and be in the moment in a completely different way. I am now an utter yogi. I crave the feelings of stillness and self-nurture that it brings – at one with myself. The old me would have probably laughed at the last sentence. But as we change and go through this new chapter, what we need in our lives will probably change too. It's just about getting to know this 'you' now.

The Calm of Restful Slumbers

Restorative slumbers form the cornerstone of a balanced perimenopausal journey. As cortisol levels fluctuate, so can our sleep patterns. Crafting a night-time ritual that fosters deep relaxation can be a beautiful way to usher in restful nights, which we so dearly need right now.

My advice would be to create a sanctuary of peace in your bedroom, with soothing hues, soft linens, and the gentle flicker of aromatic candles, crafting an ambiance that beckons restful slumbers and serene dreams.

Make sure your room is clutter-free and just feels so restful before you even think about getting into bed. Temperature is important too, so opt for slightly cooler and instead have more layers on the bed for the changing internal temperature at night.

Studies show that about 40-50% of perimenopausal women experience sleep disturbances, often linked to elevated cortisol levels.

Crafting a night-time ritual can be a wonderful strategy to foster restful slumbers during this transformative journey. See more on this in chapter 19.

Creating Your Nourishing Symphony

Nutrition plays a vital role in crafting a harmonious perimenopausal journey. Including foods rich in phytoestrogens, omega-3 fatty acids, and vibrant vegetables can create a nurturing symphony, aiding in a graceful and vibrant dance through perimenopause.

This is the best excuse now to engage in the delightful activity of crafting weekly menus that resonate with nourishment and embrace eating the rainbow. Consider integrating a vibrant array of fruits, vegetables, and lean proteins to create nutrients that supports your journey through perimenopause with more ease.

According to research published in Menopause, a journal of The North American Menopause Society, adopting a Mediterranean-style diet rich in phytoestrogens and omega-3 fatty acids significantly helped in mitigating the symptoms of perimenopause, fostering a space of vitality and balance.

See chapter 27 for more on this.

A Serenade of Self-Care

I would love you to envision crafting a personalised plan that enables you to have as much calm and serenity as possible. I promise you, my darling girl, that this is the time in your life where putting yourself first is a 'must' rather than a 'nice-to-have.'

Set aside a nurturing 'me-time' daily, immersing in activities that rejuvenate your spirit, painting, gardening, or simply watching the gentle sway of trees in the breeze, crafting moments of serene connection with your inner self. It genuinely will help you in the coming months and years.

CHAPTER 7

Be Still My Beating Heart

A candid chat about perimenopause and heart health

During perimenopause it can seem that various parts of your body engage in serious conversations about the 'changes in the weather.' This isn't always a serene gathering – sometimes it resembles an intense episode from a reality TV show. So, let's grab a comforting cup of tea (or a glass of wine, I'm not judging) and have a candid chat about how perimenopause affects the often understated yet vital communication channels in your body – specifically, the connection between your organs and your brain.

Please also see chapter 11 on gut health.

Heart Health: Cultivating a Heart-Happy Lifestyle

Isn't it about time we had a heart-to-heart about, well, heart health? Especially for women navigating the roller coaster of perimenopause and the period that follows, affectionately known as the 'beyond.'

It's hardly a secret that heart disease has an unfavourable penchant for women, becoming particularly fond of us as we journey through this chapter.

Now, before we dive into the nitty-gritty of keeping your heart bouncing happily, let's bring something crucial to light. Did you know that heart disease is the leading cause of death for women in many countries, including the UK? According to the British Heart Foundation, around 28,000 women die from a heart attack each year in the UK—that's three women every hour. Shocking right?

Now, here's where it gets tricky. The symptoms of heart disease can be different in women compared to men. While men are more likely to experience the classic chest-clutching 'Hollywood' heart attack, women might feel a broader range of symptoms—like nausea, shortness of breath, and extreme fatigue. This often leads to unfortunate misdiagnoses. In fact, studies indicate that women are 50% more likely than men to get an initial misdiagnosis after a heart attack. Yes, you read that right—50%!

Why does this matter more during perimenopause and menopause? Well, oestrogen, our hormonal BFF, tends to take a leave of absence during this period. This hormone has been our silent guardian, helping keep our blood vessels flexible and less susceptible to plaque build-up. But as oestrogen levels drop, our risk factors like high blood pressure and bad cholesterol can creep up.

So, my darling, as we wade into the waters of perimenopause, it's not just hot flushes and mood swings we need to watch out for. Our heart health needs to be top of the agenda. From lifestyle changes like healthier diets and regular exercise to medical options like hormone replacement therapy (HRT), we have various avenues to explore to keep that precious heart in tip-top shape.

There's no time like the present to invest in your heart health. After all, we're not just surviving this chapter; we're thriving through it.

Self-Help Strategies

Hormone Replacement Therapy (HRT): Embarking on the journey to protect your heart might feel like setting foot on an untrodden path. Fear not, as body identical, transdermal hormone replacement therapy (HRT) is here to hold your hand and guide you safely. There's solid evidence being whispered in the medical corridors that adopting HRT can considerably decrease the risks of heart disease. Consider this therapy your newfound ally in safeguarding your heart's fortress. More on this in later chapters.

The Role of Thoracic Flexibility: It's time to bring some twists and turns into your life, quite literally! Embracing exercises that enhance thoracic flexibility, like twists, can be a game-changer. After all, as Yamamoto and colleagues pinpointed in a 2009 study, that a flexible trunk can be a significant deterrent to arterial stiffening. So, get twisting and keep those arteries young and supple!

The Walking Charm: In this modern age, sitting has become somewhat of a chronic condition, hasn't it? But here's a golden nugget of advice: avoid marathoning those sitting sessions. Make it a point to rise and shine, take frequent walks, and stretch those limbs regularly. Your heart will thank you with a hearty beat! I have an Apple watch that nudges me every hour, but you could send a reminder on your phone or other device.

Gut Health and the Curious Connection with Constipation: The journey to a healthy heart surprisingly has a pit-stop at your gut. Yes, you read that right! Maintaining a robust gut health and preventing constipation can be your secret weapon against heart ailments. Blotcher and team in 2011, threw light on this little-known fact, indicating that preventing severe constipation can significantly reduce cardiovascular events. So, it's super important to keep things moving smoothly (see more in chapter 12 on tummy troubles).

The Power of Rest and Relaxation: In the bustling pace of life, taking moments to unwind and relax can seem like a luxury. However, incorporating practices such as yoga nidra, meditation or indulging in hypnosis recordings can be a soothing balm for your nervous system, nurturing it to foster a heart-friendly environment within you.

Sleep, Your Heart's Night-time Ally: As we already discussed, sleep is your best friend now – good news for all the sleep enthusiasts out there! Your penchant for a good night's sleep now comes with added benefits. It's proven that nurturing a healthy sleep pattern can be a formidable shield against heart diseases. So go ahead, snuggle in and dream on, for your heart is reaping the benefits with each restful minute!

The Cold-Water Chronicles: While the scientific jury might still be out deliberating, the anecdotes are pouring in favouring cold water therapy. When done correctly, immersing oneself in cold water seems to have a charm in enhancing circulation, reducing inflammation, and acting as a mood lifter. Pair this therapy with a balanced Mediterranean diet, rich in fresh food, lean meats, and whole grains, and you've got yourself a winning combination.

Exercise Your Way to a Happy Heart: Let's get those feet moving and hearts pumping with a daily dose of cardiovascular activities. Just thirty minutes of heartfelt (pun intended) exercise can be your ticket to reducing the risk of heart disease significantly. It doesn't have to be a sweaty Zumba class or a race on the treadmill, anything that significantly raises your heart rate is fabulous. Horse riding for me now is my fave – outdoors and with animals – what's not to love?

Harmonious Relationships: Believe it or not, the health of your intimate relationships has a direct bearing on your heart's wellbeing. Stress, trauma, and toxicity in relationships can potentially escalate the risk of cardiac diseases. Hence adopting non-violent communication practices can be a gateway to nurturing heart-happy relationships. See chapter 17 on relationships for more on this.

Flaxseed: In the realm of heart health, flaxseed emerges as a nutritious ally. Regular consumption of flaxseed, specifically one to two tablespoons soaked in a small amount of water, has shown promise in preventing cardiovascular diseases. It's a simple yet potent remedy to keep your heart humming happily.

As we sail through the waters of perimenopause, perimenopause, and the fascinating 'beyond,' we find ourselves at a crucial juncture where nurturing our organ health becomes paramount. Ageing gracefully is not merely a phrase; it's a conscious choice we make each day through our actions and decisions.

With each passing year, we are presented with a golden opportunity to play an active and joyful role in preserving our vital organ health. It's an exhilarating journey, peppered with learning, experiences, and personal growth. As we stand at the helm, steering the ship of our wellbeing, let us do so with enthusiasm, armed with knowledge, and a heart brimming with joy and vitality.

CHAPTER 8

Dem Bones, Dem Bones, Dem Not-So-Dry Bones

A groovy guide to robust bone health

Imagine casually bending over to pick up your morning newspaper and hearing a little 'crick' sound coming from your bones – certainly not the kind of morning music you were hoping for. In fact, it might just sound like a warning bell, signalling that it's time to start paying a bit more attention to bone health. This is especially true when we are navigating the perimenopausal phase, where osteoporosis likes to sneak in uninvited.

Osteoporosis, in simple terms, is the gradual process where bones lose their density, becoming weak and quite brittle, resembling a once-crunchy biscuit now softened in a cup of tea. This doesn't happen overnight, but slowly creeps up on you, causing mild stress fractures or even broken bones from activities as innocent as bending over or even a vigorous coughing fit.

Are You at Risk? Let's Find Out

It seems that osteoporosis has a peculiar liking for certain groups of people. Before we delve into who is particularly at risk, let's clarify something: While perimenopause seems like an exclusive club, osteoporosis isn't gender-biased and can very well affect men too.

But let's put a spotlight on the people who really need to have their guards up against this sneaky bone-thief:

1. **Perimenopausal Individuals**: Yes, once again, the perimenopausal brigade seems to bear the brunt of things. Just another little challenge to add to the mix, right?

2. **People with Extremely Low Weight**: Particularly those grappling with conditions such as hyperthyroidism, which seems to have a knack for lowering body weight and weakening bones.

3. **The Smokers' Club**: If you're lighting up frequently, be warned, as this habit is known to accelerate bone density loss.

4. **High Alcohol Consumers**: Those who have a fond relationship with a gin and tonic, or a cheeky glass of fizz, may want to reconsider the bond, as excess alcohol can be a significant perpetrator in weakening bones.

Now, you might be wondering, "How would I even know if I have osteoporosis?" It's almost like a stealthy ninja, often showing its face only when you've incurred a fracture, revealing that it had been chipping away at your bones secretly all this while. But fret not, we have a trick up our sleeve – measuring your height annually. A diminishing height could be your early warning system indicating that osteoporosis is at play. Have yourself measured every six months or so and you'll easily pick up on this.

The Diagnostic Path

If you suspect that you might be grappling with this condition, the road to diagnosis is through a DEXA scan, a specialised bone density X-ray that plays detective quite well, uncovering potential fractures before they occur and determining the rate of your bone loss.

Building Your Fortress: Preventive Measures

But, my darling, let's not wait until the scan beckons. We have the power in our hands to fortify our bones, to create a formidable fortress that stands resilient against the test of time.

Hormone Replacement Therapy (HRT) is where the building of this fortress begins. This therapy, which is body-identical and transdermal, can significantly reduce the risk of osteo-porosis. It's almost like giving your bones a protective shield, ready to combat the invading forces of bone density loss.

Please see the chapters on HRT for more information and to make an informed decision on whether or not it's right for you.

Remember that our bones are not static structures but dynamic and living tissues. They are not inert pillars but responsive entities that react to the daily choices we make. Therefore, every day is a new opportunity to strengthen our bone health.

Self-Help Strategies

Exercise: Movement is one of your powerful allies in this fight against osteoporosis. Particularly, weight-bearing exercises seem to be the superheroes here, stimulating osteoblast activity, which is essential for bone formation. When you engage in high-impact exercises or weightlifting, it's like hosting a party where osteoblasts are the guests of honour, working tirelessly to fortify your bones.

Dietary Choices: what we choose to eat can also play a starring role in this narrative. Including dark green leafy vegetables in your diet is like handing over the building blocks to these osteoblasts, providing them with the much-needed calcium to strengthen the bones. However, beware of the villains in this story – smoking, excessive alcohol, and processed foods. They are notorious for robbing your bones of calcium, diverting it to other vital organs when the deficiency strikes.

Added Supplements: To make the most out of the calcium intake, pair it with vitamin D, a dynamic duo that works wonders for your bones. You can find this combination in fortified plant milks. However, tread carefully with calcium supplements and consult with a healthcare provider before diving into supplementation, as unsupervised intake can potentially increase heart attack risks.

(You can read more about supplements in chapter 30.)

Ditch the Rennie: Regular use of antacid medicines can potentially be a contributing factor towards osteoporosis, interfering with how your body absorbs calcium. It's always best to approach stomach acid issues naturally, ensuring that the calcium you consume is put to good use.

Nurture a Healthy Gut: A happy tummy is the cornerstone of overall well-being. Improving gut health enhances the bioavailability of the food you eat and the supplements you take, thus indirectly promoting robust bone health.

See also chapter 12 on gut health.

In this chapter, we've ventured into the world of bones, uncovering the secrets to maintaining a robust skeletal system even as we age. As we wrap up, remember that your bones are living, breathing entities, constantly reshaping, and rejuvenating themselves. Every choice you make, from your diet to your daily activities, is a step towards fostering a healthy bone environment.

As you step into each day, envision yourself as the master architect of your bone fortress, meticulously crafting a structure that stands tall and unyielding, ready to support you through life's beautiful journey. Remember, as Jim Rohn once said,

"Take care of your body. It's the only place you have to live."

CHAPTER 9

Where Did I Put My Keys?

Untangling brain fog and boosting brainpower

As we gracefully age, it's not just our bodies that undergo transformations; our brains are also along for the ride. If you've ever walked into a room and forgotten why you're there, or found yourself grappling with that elusive word on the tip of your tongue, you're in good company. This chapter aims to shed light on the often-overlooked aspects of women's health during midlife: brain health, brain fog, and memory. We'll explore why these issues occur, how prevalent they are, and most importantly, what you can do about them.

Difficulty Concentrating and Memory Lapse: The Dynamic Duo

When difficulty in concentrating teams up with memory lapses, it can feel like you're battling a formidable dynamic duo in the ring of perimenopause. These two challenges often go hand-in-hand, manifesting as forgetfulness in the middle of tasks or an inability to recall names, dates, and details that you once knew like the back of your hand. A study by the University of Rochester reveals that up to 60% of women in midlife report issues with concentration and memory.

Gloria Steinem's insightful words, (that I truly love), have never been more appropriate:

"The truth will set you free, but first it will piss you off."

The comfort of knowing you're not alone in this battle comes with a sprinkle of frustration because – let's face it – you'd rather not be in this club in the first place.

So why does this dynamic duo make its grand entrance during perimenopause and menopause? The root cause is often hormonal fluctuations that have a cascading effect on your cognitive functions. Oestrogen, the hormone that begins its slow decline during this life phase, is a crucial player in managing neurotransmitters like serotonin and dopamine. These neurotransmitters act like chemical messengers, transmitting signals between nerve cells to help us focus, remember, and even regulate our mood. When oestrogen wanes, these messengers can get a little lost, leading to lapses in concentration and memory.

The ramifications can range from mild annoyances to more impactful disruptions in your day-to-day life. You might find it challenging to juggle multiple tasks at work, maintain attention during long meetings, or even keep track of personal responsibilities like bill payments or appointments. Socially, the impact can be equally disconcerting. Ever walked into a room and felt a sense of déjà vu, not because you've been there before, but because you've forgotten why you entered in the first place? Or have you ever run into someone whose name you should absolutely know, but your mind draws a blank?

Don't worry; all is not lost. This cognitive fog isn't a permanent state. There is a plethora of interventions to consider. Lifestyle adjustments such as regular exercise, mindfulness techniques, and balanced nutrition can help. Some people find relief with hormone replacement therapy (HRT), although this should only be considered after an in-depth conversation with your healthcare provider about its pros and cons (and see the chapters on The History of HRT, and HRT).

Ultimately, knowledge is your superpower against this dynamic duo. Being informed enables you to consult professionals, experiment with treatments, and find the combination of strategies that will serve as your dynamic counter-duo. Yes, it might be a formidable challenge, but remember, you're even more so.

Self-Help Strategies

Mindfulness Meditation: Studies have shown that mindfulness can improve attention and concentration. Even dedicating ten minutes a day to mindfulness can make a difference.

Physical Exercise: Regular physical activity increases blood flow to the brain, which can help improve cognitive functions. Aim for at least 150 minutes of moderate exercise per week.

Healthy Diet: Foods rich in antioxidants, good fats, and vitamins can provide an essential boost to brain health. Incorporate more fruits, vegetables, and lean proteins into your diet.

Difficulty Concentrating: The Wandering Mind

Concentration issues can be a real stumbling block during perimenopause, leaving you feeling as though your brain has decided to take a meandering stroll when you need it to run a marathon. One of the main culprits behind these difficulties is fluctuating oestrogen levels. Oestrogen plays a significant role in regulating neurotransmitters like serotonin, which, in turn, can affect your focus, attention, and overall cognitive function.

In more practical terms, you might find that tasks which once required minimal effort now demand Herculean concentration. Whether you're sifting through emails, trying to keep up with a conversation, or simply reading a book, the constant mental wandering can be disheartening.

And let's not even talk about trying to remember where you put your keys! According to research, approximately 60% of women going through perimenopause report problems with concentration.

Now, the good news is that these concentration difficulties are often temporary. However, the bad news is that they can contribute to increased stress and reduced efficiency, creating a somewhat vicious cycle. Your confidence may take a hit, leading you to question your capabilities at work or in personal pursuits, which only further exacerbates the issue.

But don't despair; this is a navigable hurdle. Lifestyle changes like proper nutrition, regular exercise, and even mindfulness techniques have shown promising results in improving concentration and mental clarity. Some women also turn to hormone replacement therapy (HRT) to mitigate the effects, but this is a route you should only consider after thorough discussion with your healthcare provider.

So, if you find yourself rereading the same sentence four times or walking into rooms and forgetting why, you're not alone – and more importantly, you're not without options. Consider this a temporary detour rather than a roadblock on your intellectual highway. With the right strategies and supports, you can reroute your focus back to its optimal path.

Self-Help Strategies
Task Management: Breaking tasks into smaller, manageable parts can make them less overwhelming. Use tools like the Pomodoro Technique to help you focus.

Scheduled Breaks: Taking short breaks during tasks can improve long-term concentration. A five-minute walk or stretch can rejuvenate your mind.

Environmental Changes: A clutter-free, quiet environment can significantly improve focus. Consider noise-cancelling headphones or soft background music to aid concentration.

Memory Lapse: The Forgetful Phenomenon

A study from Aston University found that one in three women over the age of 40 experience memory lapses to some extent. But as Maya Angelou wisely said,

> *"You may not control all the events that happen to you, but you can decide not to be reduced by them."*

Self-Help Strategies
Memory Aids: Use tools like calendars, to-do lists, and apps to keep track of tasks and appointments. Digital reminders can be a lifesaver.

Mental Exercises: Puzzles, crosswords, and other brain games can help keep your mind sharp. Dedicate a few minutes each day to these activities.

Social Interaction: Engaging in meaningful conversations and social activities can stimulate the brain. Join clubs or groups that interest you to keep your mind active.

Brain Fog: The Cloud over Clarity
According to the British Menopause Society, around 50% of women experience brain fog during perimenopause and menopause. It's like your brain decided to take a little holiday without notifying you.

Self-Help Strategies
Hydration: Dehydration can exacerbate brain fog. Aim for at least eight cups of water a day.

Sleep: Lack of sleep can contribute to brain fog. Aim for seven to eight hours of quality sleep. Consider sleep aids like lavender oil or a white noise machine.

Nutrition: Foods rich in omega-3 fatty acids can help clear up brain fog. Incorporate more fish, flaxseeds, and walnuts into your diet.

Difficulty Finding Words: The Linguistic Labyrinth

This for me, as a speaker and writer, was a biggie! I've found myself in tears before not being able to remember a simple word like 'button' or 'folder'.

Difficulty with verbal expression, particularly finding the right words, is quite a perplexing, yet common, symptom experienced during perimenopause. A study from the University of California revealed that verbal memory, including word recall, declines gradually over the course of perimenopause. This can manifest as trouble remembering names, stumbling over words, or even losing your train of thought mid-sentence. While it can be concerning and even embarrassing at times, understanding that this is a common issue can be reassuring.

The root of this issue is again largely hormonal. Fluctuating levels of oestrogen can affect various cognitive functions, including verbal memory. The brain has oestrogen receptors, and when oestrogen levels are unstable, cognitive performance, including language skills, can be affected.

Self-Help Strategies

Cognitive Exercises: Brain-training exercises can help improve cognitive functions. Word puzzles, crosswords, and other language-based games may be particularly helpful in this instance. Even reading extensively can help improve vocabulary and verbal recall.

Stay Organised: Keep lists and use apps that can assist in reminding you of tasks, names, and other important information. The less clutter there is in your mind, the easier it may be to find the words you're looking for.

The UncompliKated Perimenopause Journal and *Diary* are both great resources to help with this. You can find them on www.kategrosvenor-books.com or on Amazon.

Practice Mindfulness: Stress can exacerbate cognitive difficulties. Techniques like deep breathing and mindfulness can help you become aware of your thought processes and may make it easier to recall words.

Adequate Sleep: Lack of sleep can seriously impact cognitive function. Aim for at least seven to eight hours of quality sleep per night to keep your brain in optimal working condition.

Stay Physically Active: Physical exercise has been shown to have a positive impact on cognitive function. Aim for at least 150 minutes of moderate exercise per week to help boost your cognitive abilities, including verbal skills.

Consult a Professional: If you're finding that this symptom is particularly bothersome or interfering with your daily life, consider consulting a healthcare provider for targeted advice. They may recommend certain treatments like hormone replacement therapy (HRT) or cognitive behavioural therapy.

Ginkgo Biloba: This herb is widely used for various cognitive functions, including issues with memory and concentration. While the research is mixed, some find it helpful for improving verbal recall.

Omega-3 Fatty Acids: Known for their brain-boosting properties, omega-3s can be taken as a supplement or consumed naturally in foods like fish and flaxseeds.

Rosemary Essential Oil: Some people believe that inhaling rosemary essential oil can improve memory and concentration. While scientific evidence is limited, it may be worth a try if you're open to natural remedies.

Hydration: Believe it or not, even mild dehydration can affect your cognitive abilities. Make sure you're drinking enough water throughout the day.

In summary, difficulty with finding words during perimenopause is a frustrating but often manageable issue. With a variety of self-help strategies and natural remedies, you can take proactive steps to improve your verbal skills and navigate this linguistic labyrinth with greater ease.

**Always consult with a healthcare provider before starting any new treatment or supplement.

I think this quote is special at this point as it can be quite daunting, if not frightening, for so many of us:

> *"You gain strength, courage, and confidence by every experience in which you really stop to look fear in the face."*
> ***Eleanor Roosevelt***

Fine-Tuning Your Brain Health during Perimenopause

Picture this: you walk into a room with intent, and suddenly it seems like someone pressed the delete button on your memory. Your purpose vanishes into thin air! You can almost hear the crickets chirping in the quiet corners of your mind. Ah, the joys of 'brain fog' – an unwelcome gift from perimenopause, which sometimes feels more like a practical joke from Mother Nature herself.

In 2018, a sobering statistic surfaced: dementia was cited as the leading cause of death in the UK, as per The Alzheimer's Society. Now, before panic sets in and you start visualising a future where you forget even your favourite recipe or the punchline to your best joke, take a deep breath. There is indeed a silver lining here. It's never too late to steer the ship around and venture into the serene waters of healthy brain maintenance, especially as we navigate through the energetic tides of our 40s and 50s, a time ripe for making lifestyle changes that can pay dividends in the golden years.

Now, let's face it, we all have moments where we can't find our keys or remember the name of that movie – you know, the one with that guy from that other movie? Perimenopause seems to have a knack for amplifying these moments, thanks largely to a decline in oestrogen levels. Yes, this hormone has been moonlighting as a protector of your mental faculties all this while!

Again, a drop in oestrogen levels during perimenopause doesn't just signal the end of a woman's reproductive years. It has a significant impact on brain health, increasing our susceptibility to cognitive decline and various forms of dementia. And if you feel that the speed of your witty comebacks has declined, you're not alone. A noticeable loss of speed in communication often accompanies perimenopause, making us momentarily miss the razor-sharp repartee we once enjoyed.

However, doom and gloom aren't the names of the game here. Instead, let's focus on how we can turn the tables and maintain a sharp, vibrant mind even as we sail into the menopausal phase of life.

Self-Help Strategies

Master the Art of Learning: First in our toolkit is embracing the world of learning anew. They say you can't teach an old dog new tricks, but luckily, we're not pooches! Engaging in learning new skills or subjects can work wonders for your brain, fostering both neurogenesis and neuroplasticity, essentially giving your brain a youthful glow. Whether you decide to delve into the romantic language of French or to strum the strings of a guitar, every new skill acquired is a step towards a healthier brain.

Unlock the Secrets of Restful Sleep: Next up, we unravel the mysteries of sleep. Oh, sleep, that elusive lover who sometimes plays hard to get, especially during perimenopause! But cultivating a beautiful relationship with sleep is essential because it's during this time that your brain kicks into maintenance mode, de-toxifying itself from harmful substances like amyloid plaque, which has been linked to cognitive decline and dementia. But worry not, we'll delve deeper into the seductive art of embracing sleep in chapter 19.

Culinary Delights for a Healthy Brain: The journey to a healthy brain isn't just mental; it's deliciously culinary too! Treating your brain to a smörgåsbord of nutrients can be your secret weapon against cognitive decline. From the lush fields of spinach and kale to the vibrant hues of berries, your brain craves these daily delights. And don't forget a drizzle of that liquid gold, extra virgin olive oil, a powerhouse of monounsaturated fats that your brain adores.

Drink Up: Hydration is your brain's best friend, a loyal companion that never leaves its side. Since your brain can't store water, frequent hydration keeps it humming along happily. You might want to consider getting one of those two-litre bottles from Build Life – a constant reminder to keep the hydration flowing!

Harnessing the Power of Hormones: Now, let's talk about something that doesn't often make the headlines: testosterone. While this hormone is usually associated with men, it plays a crucial role in women's health too. Interestingly, a dash of testosterone seems to sprinkle a bit of magic on women's verbal learning and memory, according to a study by Davison and colleagues in 2011. So, it might be worth exploring how you can tap into this fountain of youth for your brain.

Blood Sugar: Maintaining a harmonious blood sugar balance is another pillar of brain health. Picture your blood sugar levels as a calm, gently flowing river, nurturing all it touches, rather than a torrential waterfall crashing down with all its might. Keeping it steady prevents cognitive issues that can arise from fluctuations.

HRT (Hormone Replacement Therapy): if available to you, can be a powerful ally in your quest for maintaining brain health. It's like sending in the cavalry to support your body during this significant transition.

Move Your Body: Lastly, we cannot forget the joyful dance of exercise, the balm of life during perimenopause. Whether you are swaying to the rhythm of a Zumba class or finding peace in the gentle flow of Tai Chi, incorporating regular exercise into your routine can keep your brain buzzing with joy.

Here's a friendly nudge from me: Start this exciting journey today, and let's defy the odds, making our golden years the time of vibrant mental acuity, humour, and wisdom. After all, as the great C.S. Lewis said,

"You are never too old to set another goal or to dream a new dream."

So, the next time you walk into a room and forget why, or struggle to find the right words, take a deep breath. Your brain might be taking you on a little detour, but with the right tools and mindset, you can steer it back on course. Remember, you're not alone, and you're certainly not without options. From lifestyle changes and cognitive exercises to medical treatments, there are multiple paths to reclaiming your mental clarity. Take proactive steps, consult healthcare professionals when needed, and most importantly, be kind to yourself during this journey.

Now, where did I put my keys again?

CHAPTER 10

Thunderbolts and Lightning, Very, Very Frightening?

Dealing with headaches, migraines, and electric shocks

I f perimenopause were a party, headaches, migraines, and electric shock-like sensations would be the uninvited guests who crash it. Just when you think you're getting a handle on hot flushes and mood swings, these symptoms arrive to add another layer of complexity.

"You are braver than you believe, stronger than you seem, and smarter than you think.
When life throws you a curveball, remember, you've got the bat!"
Kate Grosvenor

Headaches: The Common Culprit in Perimenopause

Headaches are incredibly common during perimenopause. According to the Migraine Trust, women are more than twice as likely as men to experience tension-type headaches and migraines, especially during this transitional phase.

The Causes
Hormonal Fluctuations: The ebb and flow of oestrogen during peri-menopause can trigger headaches.

Stress: The emotional roller coaster of perimenopause can lead to tension headaches.

Diet: Foods high in sugar, caffeine, or alcohol can exacerbate headaches during this period.

Self-Help Strategies

Hydration: Dehydration can worsen headaches. The traditional "aim for at least eight cups of water a day" is very outdated and doesn't take into account the differences between women. Instead, the amount of water you should drink can vary depending on your body weight and lifestyle. Here's a simple equation to give you a general idea:

Equation for Daily Water Intake:
Daily Water Intake (in litres) = (Body Weight (in kg) × 0.033) + (Life-style Factor × 0.5))

Lifestyle Factors:
- Sedentary: 0
- Lightly active (e.g., walking, light housework): 1
- Moderately active (e.g., light exercise 1-3 days a week): 2
- Very active (e.g., moderate exercise 3-5 days a week): 3
- Extremely active (e.g., vigorous exercise 6-7 days a week): 4

How to Use the Equation:
1. Multiply your body weight in kilograms by 0.033 to get your basic water needs.

2. Add additional water based on your lifestyle factor, multiplied by 0.5 litres.

Example:

Let's say you weigh 70 kg, and you are moderately active.

Daily Water Intake = (70×0.033) + (2×0.5) = 2.31 + 1 = 3.31 litres

In this example, you would aim to drink approximately 3.31 litres of water per day.

Remember, this is a general guideline and individual needs can vary. Always consult with a healthcare provider for personalised advice.

Relaxation Techniques: Deep breathing or progressive muscle relaxation can help alleviate tension headaches.

Dietary Changes: Reducing intake of trigger foods can make a significant difference during perimenopause. For me it can be chocolate and cheese (hey, I never said it was going to be fair). Take time to find out what triggers you.

Migraines: The Debilitating Dilemma of Perimenopause

Migraines are not just 'bad headaches'; they are a complex neurological condition that can be debilitating. During perimenopause, hormone fluctuations can contribute to increased frequency and severity of migraines. According to the World Health Organisation, migraines rank as the sixth highest cause of days lost due to disability worldwide. For women navigating perimenopause, the migraine dilemma can be particularly burdensome, affecting quality of life, work, and relationships.

During perimenopause, levels of oestrogen and progesterone fluctuate more erratically than usual. These hormonal shifts can affect neurotransmitter levels and blood vessels in the brain, triggering migraines or making existing ones more severe.

The Causes

Hormonal Changes: Fluctuations in hormones, particularly around the menstrual cycle, can trigger migraines.

Sensory Overload: The heightened sensitivity during perimenopause can make you more susceptible to migraine triggers like bright lights and strong smells.

Diet: Certain foods can trigger migraines, and these triggers may change or intensify during perimenopause.

Self-Help Strategies

Tracking Triggers: Understanding what sets off your migraines is the first step towards effective management. Keep a migraine diary, noting down factors like stress, foods, sleep quality, and physical activity. Look for patterns that can help you pre-emptively address triggers.

Hormone Replacement Therapy (HRT): Consult with your healthcare provider about HRT. It's not for everyone, and there are some risks to consider (though far less than the media has reported – see chapter 24 on the history of hormones) but stabilising your hormone levels could potentially reduce migraine frequency and severity.

Dietary Adjustments: Some women find that certain foods or additives can trigger migraines. Consider a diet rich in fruits, vegetables, lean protein, and whole grains. Limit intake of potential triggers like caffeine, alcohol, and artificial sweeteners.

Mindfulness and Stress Management: Stress is a well-known migraine trigger. Mindfulness techniques such as deep breathing, meditation, and even yoga can help manage stress, thereby reducing the frequency of stress-induced migraines.

Physical Activity: Moderate exercise releases endorphins, which can act as natural painkillers. However, exercise can also be a trigger for some people, so listen to your body and perhaps consult with a physiotherapist for a tailored exercise plan.

Over-the-Counter Remedies: Non-prescription options like Excedrin Migraine, Nurofen Migraine, or ibuprofen can offer relief but should be used as advised by a healthcare professional. Frequent use can lead to "rebound headaches," a nasty cycle you'll want to avoid.

Proactive Sleep Hygiene: Lack of sleep can exacerbate migraines. Aim for seven to nine hours of quality sleep per night. Keep your sleeping environment dark, quiet, and cool to encourage better sleep. See also chapter 19.

Consult a Specialist: If migraines become frequent or debilitating, it may be time to consult a headache specialist. Prescription medications and other targeted therapies could offer relief when other strategies fail.

Feverfew: Feverfew is a medicinal plant that has been used for centuries to treat headaches and migraines. The active compound, parthenolide, is thought to reduce inflammation and improve blood vessel tone. Feverfew can be consumed as a tea, a tincture, or in capsule form. I grow this on a pot on my terrace and it's easy to care for. Always consult your healthcare provider before starting any new herbal remedies, as they can interact with other medications.

Magnesium: Low magnesium levels have been linked to migraines. Consider taking magnesium supplements or including magnesium-rich foods like spinach, almonds, and bananas in your diet. Again, consult your healthcare provider for the appropriate dosage.

Peppermint Oil: Inhaling peppermint oil or applying it diluted to your temples may relieve tension and potentially reduce migraine pain. Peppermint has vaso-dilating and vaso-constricting properties, which help control blood flow in the body.

Butterbur: Another herbal remedy, butterbur is believed to have anti-inflammatory and antispasmodic effects. Some studies have suggested that butterbur can reduce the frequency of migraines, but it's essential to consult a healthcare provider for appropriate dosing and to ensure it doesn't interfere with other medications you may be taking.

Ginger: Ginger is known for its anti-inflammatory properties. Some people find relief from migraines by drinking ginger tea or taking ginger supplements. It may be particularly useful for nausea that often accompanies migraines.

Acupressure and Acupuncture: These ancient Chinese techniques aim to balance the body's energy flow by stimulating specific points. Some people find relief from migraine symptoms through acupressure or acupuncture sessions.

Lavender Oil: Inhaling the aroma of lavender essential oil may reduce symptoms of migraines. Some people find that putting a few drops of the oil on a tissue and inhaling deeply can help relieve tension and pain.

Hydration: Dehydration can be a significant trigger for migraines. Ensure you're drinking enough water, particularly if you're active or it's a hot day. A hydration tracker or regular reminders can keep you on track.

Remember, it's crucial to consult your healthcare provider before starting any natural remedies, especially if you're already taking medication or undergoing other forms of treatment.

By incorporating these natural remedies along with lifestyle changes and possibly medical treatments, you can build a comprehensive strategy for managing your perimenopausal migraines and make a significant difference.

**Always consult with your healthcare provider before beginning any new treatment.

Remember, you're not alone on this journey, and while migraines are incredibly challenging, there are steps you can take to manage the pain and reclaim your life.

Electric Shock-Like Sensations: The Jolting Experience of Perimenopause

Electric shock-like sensations, often termed as "brain zaps," are a lesser-known but equally unsettling symptom that some women experience during perimenopause. These sensations can feel like a jolt, buzz, or even a mild electric shock in the head or across other parts of the body. They can be momentary but jarring, causing a sense of disorientation or distress.

The Causes
Although the exact cause of these sensations isn't well-understood, they're thought to be linked to the fluctuating hormone levels typical of perimenopause. These shifts can affect neurotransmitter levels in the brain, leading to various neurological symptoms, including these electric shock-like sensations.

Self-Help Strategies
Journaling and Monitoring: Start by keeping a detailed journal to record when these sensations occur. Note any accompanying symptoms and potential triggers such as stress, caffeine intake, or lack of sleep. Tracking your symptoms can help identify patterns and triggers, which is valuable information for both you and your healthcare provider. *"The UncompliKated Perimenopause Journal"* is a great resource to help with this.

Stress Management Techniques: Stress can exacerbate many symptoms of perimenopause, including electric shock-like sensations. Consider stress-management techniques like deep-breathing exercises, mindfulness, and progressive muscle relaxation to keep stress at bay. Aww chapter 16 for an in-depth discussion on this.

Regular Exercise: A consistent exercise routine can help in the overall management of perimenopausal symptoms. Exercise releases endorphins, which act as natural mood stabilisers and may help mitigate the occurrence of these sensations.

Balanced Diet: Nutrient imbalances can sometimes contribute to neurological symptoms. Ensure your diet is rich in essential nutrients, particularly omega-3 fatty acids, which support brain health, and B-vitamins, known for their role in nerve function.

Consult a Healthcare Provider: Given the neurological nature of these symptoms, consulting a healthcare provider for an accurate diagnosis and tailored treatment plan is advisable.

Medication**: In some cases, medication such as hormone replacement therapy (HRT) or certain types of antidepressants may be prescribed to manage neurological symptoms during perimenopause. Always consult a healthcare provider for the treatment most suited to you.**

Omega-3 Supplements: Omega-3 fatty acids are known for their anti-inflammatory properties and their role in brain health. Some people find relief from neurological symptoms by taking omega-3 supplements.

GABA Supplements: Gamma-aminobutyric acid (GABA) is an inhibitory neurotransmitter that plays a role in calming the nervous system. Some women find that GABA supplements can help alleviate symptoms, although you should consult your healthcare provider before starting any new supplement regimen.

Herbal Teas: Herbal teas like chamomile and lavender may have calming effects on the nervous system. While not a direct treatment for electric shock-like sensations, they may contribute to overall stress reduction, thereby lessening the severity or frequency of symptoms.

Acupuncture: Though research is limited, some individuals report a reduction in neurological symptoms after acupuncture treatment. If you're open to alternative therapies, it may be worth trying.

In summary, while electric shock-like sensations during perimenopause can be distressing, a range of self-help strategies and natural remedies exist that may help you manage these symptoms. It's crucial, as always, to consult your healthcare provider before starting any new treatment, but know that you're not alone in this experience and that relief is possible.

The American Angle: A Comparative Note

In the United States, migraines affect approximately 12% of the population, and perimenopausal women are a significant subset of this group. The approach to treatment often involves a combination of medication and lifestyle changes, similar to the UK.

Headaches, migraines, and electric shock-like sensations can be incredibly disruptive, especially during perimenopause, but they don't have to control your life. With the right self-help solutions, medical advice, and lifestyle changes, you can manage these symptoms more effectively. Remember, you're not alone on this journey, and help is available. Take proactive steps, consult healthcare professionals when needed, and most importantly, be kind to yourself as you navigate the challenges of perimenopause.

CHAPTER 11

Your Overflowing Bath and How to Plug It

Histamine intolerance is a *thing*

Picture this, darlings: your body is like a luxurious bathtub, where everything should flow in perfect harmony, but sometimes, especially during perimenopause, it's like someone turned on the tap of histamine and forgot about the plug, causing a chaotic overflow. Now, before you think you're on a sinking ship, let's understand that dealing with histamine intolerance during perimenopause is much like getting to grips with a mischievous bathtub – it needs attention and a bit of finesse to keep everything in balance.

However, histamine is not all bad; it's actually a very diligent neurotransmitter, busily working in your central nervous system, digestive system, and immune system. But, like an overly enthusiastic party guest, it can overstay its welcome, causing a riot of symptoms that could have you feeling like you're hosting a full-blown fiesta inside your body.

Symptoms of Intolerance

Here's where the fun begins (or not), ladies – the grand list of symptoms you might encounter with histamine intolerance:

- A sneezing symphony after indulging in certain foods or alcohol

- Swollen hands or feet – it's not just a weird reaction to your favourite cheese!

- Itchy eyes or skin, often mistaken as your desire to flirt, winking too often

- A mosaic of hives

- The dizziness that's not from twirling in your favourite dress

- Headaches that feel like a tiny drummer playing in your head

- A nasal congestion that's frankly just not a good look

- Anxiety, racing heart, and insomnia – a cocktail of unrest

- And let's not forget post-nasal drip, tinnitus, and arrhythmia joining the party uninvited

Mary Wollstonecraft said,

"I do not wish them [women] to have power over men, but over themselves."

So, let's reclaim power over our bodies!

The science bit tells us that histamine intolerance is often a sign of high oestrogen and low DAO (diamine oxidase). During perimenopause, the progesterone that helps uplift DAO levels takes a nosedive, pushing us into a vicious cycle of histamine overload and oestrogen dominance. It's like a drama series with no end!

But fear not, the season finale is within reach. It's time to be your own hero and break this cycle. Let's face it, we've tackled worse on a Monday morning!

Self-Help Strategies

Combat Oestrogen Dominance: Be proactive in ensuring adequate progesterone levels, particularly in the latter half of your cycle. Balance is key, and it's not just about your yoga poses!

Boost Your Defence with Proper Nutrition: As in most epic tales, there are friends and foes. In our histamine story, the foes are cured meats, mature cheese, strawberries, certain wines, dried fruits, and a few veggies like spinach and tomatoes. But fret not, because our allies are just around the corner. Embrace the comforting company of lower histamine foods like rocket, cabbage, radish, watercress, and courgette. Throw in a relaxing nettle tea party, and you're on your way to victory.

Supplement Your Arsenal: Enlist the support of vitamin C with Quercetin, a DIM supplement to help with oestrogen dominance, and a DAO supplement to replenish the enzyme that breaks down histamine. (See more on supplements at the back of this book.)

Medicinal Back-up: Sometimes, we need a little extra help. Don't hesitate to consider antihistamines when the symptoms get too boisterous. Remember, it's not a sign of defeat but a strategy for winning the war.

Stress Management: Remember, darling, stress is like that unwanted party crasher. Whether it's actual or perceived, it adds to the chaos. Incorporate stress management techniques, some of which we will delve into later, to keep the party in control.

Food Avoidance: If you're concerned about histamine intolerance, you may want to be cautious with the following foods:

1. Fermented Foods: Things like sauerkraut, soy sauce, and yogurt.
2. Aged Cheeses: Such as cheddar, gouda, and camembert.
3. Processed Meats: Like salami, pepperoni, and luncheon meats.
4. Alcohol: Especially red wine, champagne, and beer.
5. Vinegar: And foods containing vinegar such as pickles.

6. Canned or Smoked Fish: Including mackerel, tuna, and sardines.
7. Vegetables: Such as tomatoes, avocados, and eggplants.
8. Dried Fruits: Apricots, prunes, dates, figs, and raisins.
9. Nuts: Especially walnuts and cashews can be high in histamine.
10. Certain Spices: Such as cinnamon, chilli powder, and cloves.
11. Strawberries

If you find you're sensitive to these foods, it's always best to consult with a healthcare provider for diagnosis and a tailored treatment plan.

So, here's to showing your strength, embracing the chaos, and turning off that histamine tap to enjoy a calm and soothing bath of wellbeing!

CHAPTER 12

Tummy Troubles and Hormonal Hubbub

The perimenopause gut connection

Perimenopause is a time of significant change, and not just in the emotional and psychological realms. Physically, many women notice shifts in their body composition, appetite, and even digestive health. As the saying goes, "Your body is a temple," but during perimenopause, it can feel more like a construction site – constantly under renovation. So, let's put on our hard hats and explore these changes, offering some strategies for managing them.

In the wondrous world of bodily functions, your gut isn't just a food-processing unit; it's a vibrant powerhouse bustling with neurotransmitters and microbes that are vested with the vital duty of maintaining balance in your body. Think of these microbes as the seasoned hosts of a daily talk show where the brain is the star guest, who are engaged in profound discussions that influence your overall health, particularly during the menopausal transition.

The Oestrobolome: Your Gut's Hormonal Maestro

You've probably heard of the gut microbiome, that bustling metropolis of microbes living in your digestive system. But have you heard of the oestrobolome? This subset of the gut microbiome is like the conductor of your hormonal orchestra, specifically focusing on the metabolism and modulation of oestrogen. When the oestrobolome is in harmony, so is your oestrogen. But when it's out of tune, you could be facing a range of oestrogen-related issues. Let's delve deeper into this fascinating topic.

The Role of the Oestrobolome

The oestrobolome is a collective name for the specific group of microbes that reside in your gut. While they are part of the larger gut microbiome, these particular bacteria have a very specialised job: they metabolise and modulate oestrogen levels in your body.

The oestrobolome produces an enzyme called beta-glucuronidase. This enzyme plays a crucial role in breaking down oestrogen so that it can be properly eliminated from the body. When this process works smoothly, your oestrogen levels are balanced, and all is well.

The Consequences of an Imbalanced Oestrobolome

Oestrogen Dominance

As we embark on this discussion, let's first acknowledge the entity that adds a touch of charm to hormones yet requires a tactful exit strategy – conjugated oestrogen. If the oestrobolome isn't functioning optimally – often due to stress, poor diet, or other lifestyle factors – oestrogen may not be broken down as it should be. Instead, it recirculates back into the bloodstream, leading to a condition known as oestrogen dominance. This can result in a variety of health issues, such as fibroids, endometriosis, and migraines.

According to a study published in the *British Journal of Nutrition*, nearly 25% of women in the UK experience gut health issues, which could potentially affect their oestrobolome and, consequently, their oestrogen levels. In the U.S., the numbers are even higher, with up to 30% of women reporting similar problems.

Ensuring a Healthy Oestrobolome

A balanced oestrobolome is crucial for hormonal harmony. That means doing everything you can to ensure good gut health is not just beneficial for digestion; it's essential for hormonal balance. It is a critical yet often overlooked component of women's health, particularly during perimenopause when hormonal fluctuations are at an all-time high. By understanding its role and taking steps to maintain a healthy gut, you can achieve hormonal harmony and mitigate a range of oestrogen-related issues. So, the next time you think about gut health, remember it's not just about digestion; it's about hormonal balance too.

Weight Gain: The Unwanted Souvenir – A Journey, Not Just Extra Pounds

According to the NHS, nearly half of women will gain weight during this phase of life. That's not just a Christmas food baby that refuses to leave; that's an entirely new you. And, of course, this phenomenon isn't exclusive to the British Isles. Stateside, around 45% of women also report gaining weight during perimenopause. So, it's safe to say, you're in expansive company!

The Causes:

Hormonal Fluctuations: Lower levels of oestrogen are like that friend who insists on ordering dessert for the table; they contribute to your weight gain even when you didn't ask for it. Reduced oestrogen levels have been shown to influence how fat is distributed in the body, often relocating it to the abdominal area.

Metabolism: Ah, metabolism, that fickle fire that once let you devour an entire pizza without a second thought. Studies show that metabolism can slow down by up to 5% per decade after you turn 40. So, the calories that used to vanish like magic now stick around like they're paying rent.

Reduced Physical Activity: As women age, lifestyle changes may result in decreased physical activity, which can contribute to weight gain. lack of energy and motivation.

Stress and Emotional Eating: Perimenopause often coincides with a stressful period in a woman's life, which can lead to emotional eating and, subsequently, weight gain. (Also see the chapter on stress for more information).

Insulin Resistance: Hormonal changes can also affect the way your body processes sugar, potentially leading to insulin resistance and weight gain. See also chapter 11.

Sleep Disorders: Conditions like insomnia or sleep apnoea can disrupt your sleep patterns, affecting the body's metabolism and leading to weight gain.

Medication: Some medications commonly taken during perimenopause for various symptoms, such as antidepressants, can have weight gain as a side effect.

Self-Help Strategies
Regular Exercise: No one is asking you to train for a marathon (unless you want to, then go you!). However, regular cardio and strength training can make a world of difference. Studies published in *Menopause*: the journal of the North American Menopause Society show that as little as thirty minutes of exercise a day can significantly counteract weight gain during perimenopause.

Balanced Diet: If your diet is mostly composed of the 'three Cs' (cake, crisps, and chocolate), it might be time for a dietary revamp (with zero judgement from me, I promise, I've been there!). Focus on foods high in protein, fibre, and healthy fats. Omega-3 fats, found in fish and flax-seeds, have been shown to assist in weight loss. Foods like avocados and lentils can also become your new best friends; they are filling and packed with nutrients.

Mindfulness and Stress Management: Mindfulness techniques and stress management strategies like deep breathing exercises or yoga can help control emotional eating.

Consult a Healthcare Provider: If you need more help. It might be helpful to consult a healthcare provider for a comprehensive plan tailored for you, which may include medication adjustments or specific dietary recommendations.

Green Tea: Research published in the *International Journal of Obesity* shows that the catechins in green tea can help burn fat. Swap your morning latte for a green tea and you're already winning.

Cinnamon: A study in the *Journal of Nutritional Science and Vitaminology* found that cinnamon can help regulate blood sugar, which in turn can help control weight. Sprinkle some on your morning porridge or use it to spice up a healthy smoothie.

Apple Cider Vinegar: While it's not a magic potion, some studies suggest that apple cider vinegar can help with weight loss. It's said to help you feel full quicker, so you eat less. Just make sure to dilute it well; you don't want to add 'burnt oesophagus' to your list of worries.

Weight gain during perimenopause can feel like you're being body-snatched by an inflated version of yourself. But remember, you have the tools and strategies to fight back. But please remember that perimenopause is a phase of life, not a life sentence. Being proactive about managing the causes of weight gain can help you navigate this period with grace and, hopefully, with your current wardrobe still in play.

The Additional Factor: Oestrogen Production Beyond the Ovaries

Interestingly, your ovaries aren't the only part of your body that produces oestrogen. Fat cells can also produce this hormone, which adds another layer of complexity to the weight gain issue. As your ovaries slow down their oestrogen production during perimenopause, your body might try to compensate by holding onto more fat cells, essentially creating an alternative oestrogen source. This can create a bit of a vicious cycle: lower oestrogen levels lead to weight gain, and the additional fat cells then produce more oestrogen. It's like your body's own version of a catch-22, but with more hormonal drama.

This additional factor underscores the importance of managing weight gain during perimenopause. It's not just about aesthetics or fitting into your favourite pair of jeans; it's also about hormonal balance and overall health. So, while weight gain during this phase may be common, understanding the multiple factors at play can empower you to take proactive steps in managing it.

The Waist-Hip Ratio: More Than Just a Number

Many women report a noticeable change in their waist-hip ratio during perimenopause, with a shift in weight distribution that favours the midsection. While you might initially be concerned about how this affects your silhouette or the fit of your favourite skirt, the implications go far beyond aesthetics. This change in body composition is not just a cosmetic issue; it's a significant health concern that warrants attention.

The shift in weight to the abdominal area is often due to hormonal changes, primarily the decrease in oestrogen levels. Oestrogen has a role in determining where fat is stored in the body, and as its levels decline, you're more likely to see fat accumulate around the abdomen rather than the hips or thighs. This is often referred to as the 'middle-age spread,' but don't let the casual name fool you; it's a phenomenon that has serious health implications.

The Health Risks of Abdominal Fat

Abdominal fat is not just any fat; it's a specific type known as visceral fat, which is stored deep inside the abdominal cavity and surrounds vital organs like the liver and pancreas. Unlike subcutaneous fat, which sits just under the skin, visceral fat is metabolically active and can release fatty acids and inflammatory agents into the bloodstream. This can lead to a host of health issues, including:

Cardiovascular Disease: Visceral fat is linked to higher levels of LDL cholesterol ('bad' cholesterol) and lower levels of HDL cholesterol ('good' cholesterol), increasing the risk of heart disease.

Insulin Resistance: The fatty acids released by visceral fat can lead to insulin resistance, a precursor to type 2 diabetes.

Inflammation: The inflammatory agents released can contribute to a state of chronic inflammation, which is linked to a range of health issues from arthritis to cancer.

Self-Help Strategies

Understanding the health risks associated with a changing waist-hip ratio can be empowering rather than frightening. It gives you the information you need to take proactive steps to manage this aspect of perimenopause. Strategies can include:

Regular Exercise: Cardiovascular exercise can help burn fat, while strength training can increase muscle mass, boosting your metabolism.

Dietary Changes: A balanced diet rich in whole grains, lean protein, and healthy fats can help manage weight. Reducing sugar and processed foods is also beneficial.

Stress Management: High stress levels can lead to weight gain, particularly in the abdominal area. Stress management techniques like deep breathing, meditation, and even short walks can help.

In summary, a changing waist-hip ratio during perimenopause is not just a matter of needing a new wardrobe. It's a sign of underlying physiological changes that can have significant health implications. By understanding what's happening and why, you can take steps to manage your health proactively.

Bloating: The Inflatable You, Unveiled

Bloating during perimenopause is so common that it could almost be considered a rite of passage. According to a study published in the journal *Menopause*, a staggering 70% of women experience bloating during this transitional phase. That's more than two-thirds of women who are navigating the perimenopausal journey. And we're not talking about a slight puffiness that can be easily ignored; for many, the bloating can be intense enough to interfere with daily activities, wardrobe choices, and even relationships. It's not just an inconvenience; it's a significant concern that can impact your quality of life.

The Causes

So, what's behind this bloating? It's not as if you've suddenly turned into a human balloon. Several factors contribute to this uncomfortable symptom:

Hormonal Fluctuations: The hormonal changes that occur during perimenopause can affect your digestive system. Lower levels of oestrogen can slow down the gastrointestinal tract, leading to bloating and even constipation.

Dietary Choices: Certain foods are known to cause bloating, such as beans, lentils, carbonated drinks, and certain vegetables like broccoli and cauliflower. Your digestive system may become more sensitive to these foods during perimenopause.

Water Retention: Hormonal changes can also lead to water retention, which can make you feel bloated. This is particularly common in the days leading up to your period.

Stress: Believe it or not, stress can also contribute to bloating. Stress hormones can affect gut motility and contribute to gastrointestinal issues.

The Health Implications
While bloating itself is generally not a serious health concern, it can be a symptom of other underlying issues, such as irritable bowel syndrome (IBS) or food intolerances. Persistent bloating should be evaluated by a healthcare provider to rule out more serious conditions.

Self-Help Strategies
Understanding the root causes of bloating can empower you to take steps to manage it. Here are some things you can do to help yourself:

Dietary Changes: Keep a food diary to identify foods that trigger bloating and consider eliminating them from your diet. Opt for foods that are easier on the digestive system, like bananas, cucumbers, and ginger.

Hydration: Drinking plenty of water can help reduce water retention and alleviate bloating. Aim for at least eight 8-ounce glasses a day, more if you're active but see pages 46-47 for an equation to figure out how much water would be optimal for you.

Physical Activity: Regular exercise can help keep your digestive system moving, reducing the likelihood of bloating and constipation.

Stress Management: Techniques like deep breathing, meditation, and mindfulness can help manage stress, which in turn can alleviate bloating.

THE UNCOMPLIKATED GUIDE TO PERIMENOPAUSE

Consult a Healthcare Provider: If bloating becomes a persistent issue, it may be wise to consult a healthcare provider for a thorough evaluation and tailored treatment plan.

In summary, while bloating during perimenopause may be common, it's not something you have to simply endure. With a bit of knowledge and proactive management, you can deflate the "inflatable you" and navigate this phase with greater comfort and ease.

Gut Dysbiosis

Navigating through perimenopause can sometimes feel akin to steering a ship through choppy waters. One minute it's smooth sailing, and the next, you might find yourself faced with the stormy seas of gut dysbiosis.

This complex issue occurs when the tight junctions between the cells of the gut lining slacken, commonly referred to as 'leaky gut'. This allows particles of undigested food and unmetabolised oestrogen (among other hormones) to infiltrate the bloodstream, potentially leading to inflammatory symptoms like headaches and joint pain.

Unfortunately, many women in the UK experience these symptoms, with a study indicating that up to 70% have encountered at least one digestive issue, such as bloating or irritable bowel syndrome (IBS), which are closely related to gut dysbiosis. This problem can be ignited by various factors including chronic stress, medications, and deficiencies in vital nutrients like vitamins A and D, and zinc.

However, don't fret!

"Success is not about climbing up the ladder, it is about how fulfilling and meaningful is this life I am creating. And the quality of our inner life really affects the quality of our outer life. Success is about how we can have a flourishing life, living life with a sense of well-being and of course,

health is a big part of it, wisdom, wonder and giving."
Arianna Huffington

With some diligence and proactiveness, there are straightforward strategies you can employ to maintain a healthy gut, especially during the menopausal phase.

Self-Help Strategies

Embrace Diaphragmatic Breathing: Belly breathing exercises not only enhances vagal tone but also induces relaxation in the gut's enteric nervous system. This is a simple yet effective method to nurture your gut health.

Nourish Your Good Bacteria: Incorporating prebiotic foods like leeks, garlic, ginger, soaked oats, and fermented foods into your diet can foster a healthy environment for beneficial bacteria in your gut.

Avoid Feeding the Bad Bacteria: Try to limit the intake of excessive sugar, gluten, and dairy in your diet, which can fuel harmful bacteria, exacerbating gut issues.

Consider Probiotics Wisely: Probiotics can be a great ally, but it's crucial to choose the right ones. Undertaking private testing can help pinpoint the exact type of gut flora beneficial for you, preventing any adverse effects from incorrect supplementation.

Embrace Relaxing Activities: Remember that nurturing your mind is equally important as caring for your gut. Engage in tranquil activities like yoga or Tai Chi to manage stress levels. Audrey Hepburn once advised, "To plant a garden is to believe in tomorrow." So, cherish the present moment and look forward to a brighter, healthier future.

Personalise Your Nutrition: Trust in the expertise of a nutritionist or dietitian to help carve out a nutrition plan that suits you perfectly. This strategy could be your secret weapon in identifying and avoiding foods that don't agree with your system.

Keep a Food Diary: Why not start maintaining a food diary? It can be a powerful tool, helping you track your eating patterns and pinpoint any foods that might be triggering uncomfortable symptoms.

Indulge in Gentle Exercises: Remember, a little physical activity goes a long way. Simple joys like walking or cycling can not only brighten your day but also bring harmony to your gut.

Hydrate, Hydrate, Hydrate: Keep that water bottle handy, ladies! Consistent hydration throughout the day can be a boon for your digestive system.

Discover the Comfort of Herbal Teas: Have you tried soothing herbal teas like peppermint or ginger? They might just be the comforting hug your gut needs.

Practice Mindful Eating: Let's make mealtimes a tranquil experience. Take time to savour each bite, chewing thoroughly to ease the workload on your digestive system.

Seek Support and Share: You're not alone on this journey. Consider joining support groups or therapy sessions where you can share your experiences and learn from others navigating similar paths. You are more than welcome to join my support group on Facebook 'Perimenopause with Kate Grosvenor'.

Prioritise Quality Sleep: A restful night's sleep can be a game-changer in managing gut dysbiosis. Establish a serene bedtime routine to ensure your sleep is both deep and restorative.

Embrace Positive Affirmations: Let's infuse our daily routine with positive affirmations. A positive mindset can sometimes work wonders in reducing the stress associated with gut dysbiosis. Also look at the chapter on stress and perimenopause for more effective stress management exercises and advice.

I love this inspiring and beautiful quote:

> *"My mission in life is not merely to survive, but to thrive; and to do so with some passion, some compassion, some humour, and some style."*
> **Maya Angelou**

Ladies, let's embrace this vibrant approach to life, nurturing our bodies with grace and joy at every step.

CHAPTER 13

The Softening Edges

Navigating your body's new layout with grace

During perimenopause, you might notice that your body is going through a bit of a metamorphosis, and not necessarily the kind that turns you into a butterfly. Your body composition, specifically the ratio of muscle to fat, can undergo significant changes. You may find that you're losing muscle mass while gaining fat, even if the number on the scales remains stubbornly the same. This isn't some optical illusion or a trick of the light; it's a real physiological change that many women experience.

So, what's driving this transformation? Several factors are at play.

The Causes

Hormonal Changes: Lower levels of oestrogen can affect how your body distributes fat, leading to a decrease in muscle mass and an increase in fat storage. This is particularly true for visceral fat, the type that's stored in the abdomen.

Metabolic Rate: As we age, our metabolic rate naturally slows down. A slower metabolism means you burn fewer calories at rest, which can lead to muscle loss and fat gain if you don't adjust your activity levels or calorie intake.

Reduced Physical Activity: Let's face it, life gets busy, and sometimes exercise falls by the wayside. Reduced physical activity can exacerbate the loss of muscle mass.

Nutritional Factors: Inadequate protein intake can also contribute to muscle loss, especially if you're not engaging in regular strength training.

Changes in body composition aren't just a cosmetic concern; they have real health implications. Loss of muscle mass can lead to reduced strength and mobility, making you more susceptible to falls and injuries. Increased fat, particularly visceral fat, is associated with a higher risk of cardiovascular disease, type 2 diabetes, and certain cancers.

Self Help Strategies

Understanding these changes can empower you to take proactive steps to manage them. Here are some things you can do to help yourself:

Strength Training: Incorporating strength training exercises into your routine can help you maintain or even build muscle mass. Aim for at least two sessions a week focusing on major muscle groups.

Cardiovascular Exercise: While strength training is crucial for maintaining muscle mass, don't neglect cardiovascular exercise, which is essential for heart health and weight management.

Nutrition: Make sure you're getting enough protein to support muscle maintenance. Protein-rich foods like lean meats, fish, eggs, and legumes can be excellent choices.

Caloric Intake: Be mindful of your caloric intake. Eating more calories than you burn will lead to weight gain, but eating too few can result in muscle loss.

Consult a Healthcare Provider: If you're concerned about changes in your body composition, it may be helpful to consult a healthcare provider for a thorough evaluation and tailored advice.

Changes in body composition during perimenopause are a common but manageable issue. With the right knowledge and strategies, you can navigate this shape-shifting phase of life with confidence and grace.

Changes in Appetite: The Hunger Games

The increase in appetite during perimenopause can be perplexing, especially if you've had a relatively stable appetite up until this point. Several factors contribute to this phenomenon.

The Causes

Hormonal Fluctuations: Hormones like ghrelin, known as the 'hunger hormone,' can increase during perimenopause. Ghrelin signals to your brain that it's time to eat, and if you have more of it circulating in your system, you're likely to feel hungrier more often.

Emotional Eating: The emotional roller coaster of perimenopause, including mood swings, anxiety, and depression, can lead to emotional eating. Food can be a source of comfort, and you might find yourself reaching for snacks more often as a way to cope with emotional turbulence.

Metabolic Changes: As you age, your metabolism slows down, which paradoxically can make you feel hungrier. Your body might be signalling for more food as a way to boost energy levels, even though your slower metabolism means you don't actually need the extra calories.

Blood Sugar Fluctuations: Hormonal changes can also affect insulin sensitivity, leading to fluctuations in blood sugar levels. When your blood sugar drops, you'll feel hungry, even if you've eaten recently.

Sleep Disruptions: Perimenopause often comes with sleep issues, like insomnia or poor-quality sleep, which can affect the hormones that regulate hunger and fullness, leading to increased appetite.

Understanding these factors can help you manage your increased appetite more effectively. It's not about willpower; it's about understanding the physiological and emotional changes that are affecting your eating habits. Armed with this knowledge, you can take steps to manage your appetite in a way that supports your overall well-being.

According to a survey by the British Menopause Society, 40% of women reported an increase in appetite during perimenopause. That's nearly half of the perimenopausal population suddenly feeling like they could eat a horse (not literally, of course).

Self-Help Strategies

Mindful Eating: Pay attention to what and when you eat. Instead of munching mindlessly, try to savour each bite. This helps you become more attuned to your body's hunger and fullness signals, effectively helping you eat only as much as you need.

Portion Control: Measure your servings and stick to the recommended portion sizes. By reducing portion sizes, you can still enjoy a variety of foods without overeating. Sometimes a smaller plate can trick the mind into thinking it's had enough, I know that it works for me.

Hydrate Before You Masticate: Sometimes thirst disguises itself as hunger. Drinking a glass of water before a meal can help you differentiate between thirst and genuine hunger and may also make you feel fuller, reducing the likelihood of overeating.

Eat Slowly: It takes about twenty minutes for the stomach to signal the brain that it's full. So, eat slowly and give your brain time to catch up with your stomach.

High-Protein, Low-Carb: Studies have shown that a diet higher in protein and lower in carbohydrates can help control hunger. Protein takes longer to digest, helping you feel full for longer.

Regular Exercise: Not only does exercise help you burn calories, but it also can act as an appetite suppressant. According to the Mayo Clinic, aerobic exercise is most effective in controlling appetite.

Healthy Snacks: If you're a snack girl like me, opt for healthy choices like carrot sticks, apple slices, or a handful of almonds. A study published in the European Journal of Clinical Nutrition found that almond consumption reduced hunger and the desire to eat.

Fibre is Your Friend: High-fibre foods like vegetables, fruits, and whole grains take longer to digest and thus keep you full for a longer time. The American Heart Association suggests aiming for at least twenty-five grams of fibre each day. See chapter 27 on lifestyle.

Avoid Sugary Drinks and Alcohol: Sugary drinks can cause rapid spikes in blood sugar levels, leading to a crash that will make you feel hungry again. Alcohol, on the other hand, can lower your inhibitions, making it easier to overeat.

Stay Occupied: Sometimes we eat not because we're hungry, but because we're bored. Engage in activities that divert your attention away from food.

Plan Your Meals: Having a meal plan takes the guesswork out of eating and helps you stick to a balanced diet. When you know what you're going to eat, you're less likely to 'wing it' and then become tempted by unhealthier choices that are perhaps more convenient.

Limit Stress: Elevated stress levels can release the hormone cortisol, which may lead to cravings and overeating. Techniques like deep breathing, meditation and yoga can help manage stress.

Consult a Nutritionist: For a tailored approach, consider consulting a registered nutritionist who can help create a personalised diet plan for you.

Journal Your Journey: Track what you eat and how you feel when you eat it. Noticing a pattern can help you identify emotional triggers or times when you are most likely to overeat.

Listen to Your Body: Sometimes the body just needs rest, not food. Check in with yourself; maybe that feeling of hunger is actually fatigue.

With these self-help strategies in your toolkit, navigating the realm of increased appetite during perimenopause could become a more manageable feat. And remember, while it might seem like your appetite has a mind of its own, with a little self-awareness and the right strategies, you're still the one in charge.

Food Cravings: The Siren's Call

Food cravings during perimenopause are as common as rain in the UK – almost inevitable and sometimes intense. Chocolate, sweets, and salty snacks often top the list of most-craved items. According to a survey by the British Menopause Society, a staggering 90% of respondents reported experiencing mood changes, and within that group, food cravings were a top complaint. So, if you find yourself suddenly yearning for a bar of chocolate or a bag of crisps, rest assured you're in good (and likely hungry) company.

The Causes

So, what's behind these cravings? It's not just a matter of a sweet tooth suddenly going rogue. Several factors contribute to the uptick in food cravings during perimenopause:

Hormonal Fluctuations: The hormonal roller coaster of perimenopause can affect neurotransmitters like serotonin, which regulate mood and appetite. Lower serotonin levels can lead to cravings for carbohydrates, which temporarily boost serotonin.

Emotional Eating: The emotional ups and downs that come with perimenopause can lead to emotional eating. Comfort foods, often high in sugar and fat, can provide a temporary emotional lift.

Nutritional Deficiencies: Sometimes, cravings can be your body's way of signalling a nutritional need. For example, craving chocolate could indicate a magnesium deficiency

Blood Sugar Levels: Hormonal changes can also affect insulin sensitivity, leading to blood sugar spikes and crashes, which in turn can trigger cravings for quick sources of energy like sugary snacks.

While indulging in a craving occasionally won't derail your health, frequent indulgences can add up. Excess sugar and salt can lead to weight gain, high blood pressure, and increased risk of heart disease. Not to mention, frequent sugar spikes can lead to insulin resistance, a precursor to type 2 diabetes.

Self-Help Strategies
Understanding the root causes of your cravings can help you manage them more effectively. Here are some self-help strategies:

Healthy Substitutes: Craving something sweet? Opt for fruit or a small piece of dark chocolate instead of a sugary dessert. If it's salt you're after, try air-popped popcorn seasoned with herbs.

Mindfulness: Before you reach for that snack, pause and assess your emotional state. Are you truly hungry, or are you bored, stressed, or sad? Sometimes a glass of water or a quick walk can diminish a craving.

Balanced Diet: Eating a balanced diet rich in protein, fibre, and healthy fats can help stabilise blood sugar levels, reducing the frequency of cravings.

Consult a Nutritionist: If you find that your cravings are persistent and hard to manage, it might be helpful to consult a nutritionist who can help you identify any nutritional deficiencies and recommend a balanced diet.

So, while food cravings during perimenopause may be common, they're not inevitable. With a bit of understanding and some proactive strategies, you can navigate this aspect of perimenopause without falling prey to every culinary siren call.

Digestive Problems: The Internal Rebellion Decoded

If you find yourself dealing with digestive issues during perimenopause, you're far from alone. According to the NHS, up to 60% of women experience some form of digestive discomfort during this transitional phase. That's more than half of all women navigating the perimenopausal journey. And these aren't just minor tummy troubles; for many, the symptoms can be disruptive enough to interfere with daily activities and overall well-being. Clearly, this is a pressing issue that warrants more attention and understanding.

The Causes

So, what's behind this internal rebellion? It's not as if your digestive system has suddenly decided to mutiny. Several factors contribute to these digestive issues:

Hormonal Fluctuations: The hormonal changes that occur during perimenopause can have a significant impact on your digestive system. Lower levels of oestrogen can affect gut motility, leading to symptoms like bloating, constipation, or even diarrhoea.

Stress: The emotional ups and downs that come with perimenopause can also take a toll on your digestive system. Stress hormones like cortisol can affect gut motility and contribute to symptoms like bloating and indigestion.

Dietary Choices: Your digestive system may become more sensitive to certain foods during perimenopause, exacerbating symptoms. Foods high in fat, sugar, or spice may become more difficult to digest.

Lifestyle Factors: Lack of exercise and poor hydration can also contribute to digestive issues, leading to symptoms like constipation.

While digestive issues themselves are generally not life-threatening, they can be a symptom of other underlying conditions, such as irritable bowel syndrome (IBS), food intolerances, or even gastrointestinal disorders like Crohn's disease. Persistent digestive issues should be evaluated by a healthcare provider to rule out more serious conditions.

Self-Help Strategies

Understanding the root causes of your digestive discomfort can empower you to take steps to manage it effectively. Here are some strategies:

Dietary Changes: Consider keeping a food diary to identify potential triggers and discuss it with a healthcare provider or a nutritionist. They can help you develop a diet plan that minimises digestive discomfort.

Hydration: Adequate hydration can aid in digestion and alleviate symptoms like constipation. Aim for at least eight 8-ounce glasses of water a day, more if you're active.

Regular Exercise: Physical activity can help keep your digestive system functioning smoothly. Even a short, daily walk can make a difference.

Stress Management: Techniques like deep breathing, meditation, and mindfulness can help manage stress, which in turn can alleviate digestive symptoms.

Consult a Healthcare Provider: If digestive issues become persistent or severe, consult a healthcare provider for a thorough evaluation and tailored treatment plan.

Digestive issues during perimenopause are common but manageable. With the right knowledge and proactive strategies, you can quell the internal rebellion and navigate this phase with greater digestive peace.

Also, see chapter 12 on gut health.

Diarrhoea: The Runaway Issue During Perimenopause

Diarrhoea might not be the first symptom that comes to mind when you think of perimenopause, but for some women, it's a significant and often overlooked issue. Beyond the inconvenience and discomfort, diarrhoea can lead to dehydration and nutrient loss, which can be particularly concerning during a life stage already fraught with physiological changes.

The Causes

Diet: Foods high in fat, lactose, or artificial sweeteners can be common triggers for diarrhoea.

Stress: A study published in the journal *Gastroenterology* indicates that stress can significantly impact gut health, potentially leading to issues like diarrhoea.

Hormonal Fluctuations: The hormonal changes experienced during perimenopause can affect gut motility, leading to symptoms like diarrhoea.

Self-Help Strategies

Hydration: Rehydrating is crucial when experiencing diarrhoea. The World Health Organisation (WHO) recommends oral rehydration solutions, available at pharmacies, to effectively replace lost fluids and electrolytes.

Dietary Changes: Keep a food diary to identify potential triggers. Common culprits include dairy, high-fat foods, and certain types of artificial sweeteners.

Fibre Intake: Soluble fibre found in foods like oats, beans, and certain fruits can help absorb excess water in the intestines and may alleviate diarrhoea.

Probiotics: These can restore healthy gut bacteria, potentially improving diarrhoea. A review in the *Journal of Clinical Gastroenterology* found that certain probiotics can be effective in treating various forms of diarrhoea.

Consult a Professional: If diarrhoea becomes chronic or is affecting your quality of life, it might be time to consult a healthcare provider for a comprehensive treatment plan, which may include medications like antidiarrheal agents or even hormone replacement therapy to stabilise hormonal fluctuations.

Ginger Tea: Known for its anti-inflammatory and digestive benefits, ginger tea can soothe the digestive tract.

Chamomile Tea: Its antispasmodic properties can help with intestinal cramping which often accompanies diarrhoea.

Peppermint Oil: Some studies suggest peppermint oil can relieve symptoms of irritable bowel syndrome (IBS), including diarrhoea. Enteric-coated peppermint oil capsules are usually recommended to avoid heartburn.

Bananas: Rich in pectin, a type of soluble fibre that helps absorb liquid in the intestines.

Apple Cider Vinegar: Although scientific evidence is limited, some people find that a tablespoon of apple cider vinegar in a large glass of water can provide relief from diarrhoea.

While diarrhoea during perimenopause can be an embarrassing and inconvenient issue, a range of self-help solutions and natural remedies exist that may help you manage this runaway problem effectively. Always consult your healthcare provider for diagnosis and treatment, especially before starting any new supplement or natural remedy.

Abdominal Pain: The Gut-Wrenching Experience of Perimenopause

Abdominal pain during perimenopause can be an ambiguous but distressing issue. While exact statistics are scarce, anecdotal evidence and medical observations suggest that a significant number of women face this challenge. Whether it's mild discomfort or sharp, intense pain, the experience can significantly impact your quality of life.

The Causes

Digestive Issues: Conditions like irritable bowel syndrome (IBS) can flare up or even develop for the first time during perimenopause. A study published in the *World Journal of Gastro-enterology* notes a higher prevalence of IBS symptoms among perimenopausal women.

Hormonal Fluctuations: Your gut has hormone receptors, and changes in hormone levels can impact gut motility and sensitivity, contributing to abdominal pain.

Self-Help Strategies

Pain Management: Over-the-counter medications like antispasmodics or nonsteroidal anti-inflammatory drugs (NSAIDs) can be effective for immediate relief. Always consult a health-care provider for appropriate dosages and drug interactions.

Dietary Modifications: Keeping a food diary can help identify triggers. A low FODMAP diet is often recommended for IBS-related abdominal pain.

Physical Activity: Exercise can improve digestion and alleviate stress, which could be beneficial in managing abdominal pain. According to a study in the *American Journal of Gastro-enterology*, regular physical activity can significantly improve IBS symptoms.

Stress Management: Stress can exacerbate abdominal pain. Techniques like deep breathing, meditation, and mindfulness have been shown to reduce symptoms in some individuals.

Consult a Healthcare Provider: If the abdominal pain is persistent or severe, consulting a healthcare provider for a proper diagnosis and treatment plan is essential. This could include diagnostic tests and possibly hormone replacement therapy (HRT).

Peppermint Tea: Known for its antispasmodic properties, peppermint tea can relieve abdominal cramping.

Ginger: This root has anti-inflammatory and gastrointestinal tract-soothing properties. Ginger tea or even fresh ginger in your meals can be beneficial. I quite like crystallised ginger too.

Chamomile Tea: This herb can help relax muscle spasms in the gastrointestinal tract, thus providing relief from abdominal pain.

Fennel Seeds: These seeds have antispasmodic and anti-inflammatory properties and can be chewed or steeped in hot water for a soothing tea.

Aloe Vera Juice: Some people find relief from digestive issues through aloe vera juice, which is known for its anti-inflammatory properties. However, consult your healthcare provider before trying this remedy, especially if you're taking other medications.

Abdominal pain can be a particularly gut-wrenching experience during perimenopause, but there are various self-help strategies and natural remedies that might offer relief. Always consult your healthcare provider for a comprehensive treatment plan tailored to your needs.

CHAPTER 14

The Vagina Monologue

Let's talk sex, leaks, and everything down under

We come to a chapter that may make you blush a tad but is extremely important to discuss openly – the fascinating tale of your vagina, the vibrant dance of sex, and the sometimes-unwelcome urinary concerts.

Stress Incontinence

Our bodies might start playing a few tricks on us, with stress incontinence being one of the lead jesters. Essentially, it's like your bladder develops a little sense of humour, offering you unexpected sprinkles when you laugh, cough, or even sneeze.

These little 'sprinkles of joy' happen because the muscles that support the bladder are taking it easy, perhaps too easy, during this time. But fear not, engaging in pelvic floor exercises can be a great counteraction, helping to keep those muscles in tip-top shape. Remember, a little giggle with

THE UNCOMPLIKATED GUIDE TO PERIMENOPAUSE

a sprinkle can sometimes light up your day, but keeping those muscles trained is a step towards reclaiming control.

Or it could be that sudden urge to visit the loo that seems to be happening all too often. Your bladder seems to be on high alert, ready to spring into action at a moment's notice. Again, the hormonal fluctuations are stirring the pot, making your bladder a bit more sensitive. To navigate this, try reducing irritants in your diet and practising bladder training exercises to regain control over your urinary schedule.

Embarking further into the realms of urinary incontinence, there comes a moment when we must have a candid chat about the **solutions** that have our backs, or rather our bottoms, in these times. Now, it might seem a bit daunting at first, but embracing the existence of pads and leak-proof knickers can be a real game-changer.

Imagine being able to laugh heartily, sneeze unexpectedly, or even break into an impromptu jig without a worry in the world. That's right! The modern world has blessed us with products that allow us to enjoy these simple pleasures without holding back. Leak-proof knickers are the unsung heroes in our perimenopausal journey, offering us not just protection but also an unbridled freedom to enjoy life to the fullest. These fabulous innovations come in various styles and comfort levels, ensuring that every woman finds her perfect match. See the resources section at the end of this book for my recommendations.

Moreover, let's not shy away from celebrating the humble pads that stand guard, offering security and comfort. In this period of transformation, they serve as trusty sidekicks, allowing us to navigate our daily routines with confidence and peace of mind. And what's more, they have evolved to be incredibly discreet and comfortable, adapting perfectly to our dynamic lifestyles. So, whether you're conquering the boardroom, exploring the great outdoors, or enjoying a laughter-filled evening with your friends, know that you're well-supported in every endeavour.

The Urinary Tract

Urinary issues might decide to join the party too, making their presence felt more frequently. Hormonal changes are, once again, the usual suspects, influencing the urinary tract's function. The changes might mean more frequent trips to the loo, sometimes with a sense of urgency.

Maintaining a healthy weight and avoiding irritants like caffeine and alcohol can be your golden tickets to keeping these issues at bay.

Urinary tract infections might make an appearance due to the changes in the vaginal flora and pH levels. It's vital to stay hydrated, maintain impeccable hygiene, and consult with your healthcare provider if UTIs start becoming frequent visitors.

The Midnight Tinkles

Maybe that's not as annoying as night-time trips to the loo under the moon's soft glow. They disrupt sleep and may prevent you from falling back to sleep quickly. Keeping fluids to a minimum in the evening and avoiding caffeine can sometimes help to lessen the frequency, and also try eating a small protein snack before bed.

Let's unpack why indulging in a protein snack before nestling into your sheets might just give you a night of uninterrupted slumber, sans the pesky midnight bathroom trips.

Firstly, the science behind this lies in the nature of protein itself. Consuming a protein-rich snack can potentially stabilise blood sugar levels. When blood sugar levels take a dip during the night, the body responds by producing a hormone called glucagon to increase them. This process can stimulate the kidneys to produce urine, thereby possibly increasing the likelihood of nocturnal bathroom visits. A protein snack before bedtime can provide a slower, steadier release of glucose, which might prevent the significant dips in blood sugar levels and thereby reduce the need for these middle-of-the-night bathroom excursions.

Furthermore, having a balanced blood sugar level while you are in the arms of Morpheus can promote a deeper, more restful sleep. We're talking less tossing, turning, and fewer instances of being rudely awakened by the pressing need to visit the loo. A win-win situation, you'd agree!

In addition, protein takes a bit longer to digest compared to carbohydrates. This means your body works a bit harder (burns more calories) and a bit longer to digest protein, which can help you feel fuller for a longer period and might deter the need for a midnight snack accompanied by a drink – a known culprit for nocturnal bathroom visits.

Now, before you rush to stock up your pantry with protein-rich snacks, it's worth mentioning that moderation is key here. Opt for a light snack rather than a full-fledged protein feast to avoid any potential discomfort or digestive issues during the night.

You might consider incorporating snacks such as a small handful of nuts, a piece of cheese, or a hard-boiled egg into your pre-bedtime routine. Not only are these delightful choices rich in protein, but they also contain essential nutrients that can nourish your body.

To sum up, incorporating a protein snack before bedtime is akin to giving yourself a night of serene, uninterrupted slumber, without the frantic midnight dashes to the bathroom. So go ahead, make this small tweak in your nightly routine and embrace the possibility of a blissful, undisturbed night's rest. Sweet dreams!

Vaginal Dryness

Vaginal dryness might decide to enter the scene, bringing a bit of discomfort along with it. This dry spell is primarily due to decreasing oestrogen levels. But fear not, as there are excellent lubricants and moisturisers ready to come to the rescue, turning the dry spell into a lush oasis of comfort once again.

Vaginal Atrophy

Vaginal atrophy, also known as atrophic vaginitis, tends to become a more frequent visitor as women embark on the journey of perimenopause. This condition is essentially characterised by the thinning, drying, and inflammation of the vaginal walls, which is attributed to the decline in oestrogen levels.

To understand the breadth of this phenomenon, let's bring some numbers into the picture. According to various studies, approximately 50% of postmenopausal women will experience symptoms of vaginal atrophy, although it can start manifesting during the perimenopausal phase. However, the striking fact here is that only about 20-25% of women seek medical help to address these symptoms, indicating that a significant portion of women endure these changes silently, without seeking the potential relief and support available.

The stage is primarily set by the waning levels of oestrogen in the body, a hormone that has been playing a pivotal role in maintaining the health and elasticity of vaginal tissues. As oestrogen takes a bow, the vaginal tissue becomes thinner, less elastic, and more fragile, making it more susceptible to injury and infection.

The beauty of this phase is that with awareness and proactive measures, it's entirely possible to combat the symptoms of vaginal atrophy and maintain a fulfilling and comfortable sexual life.

Self-Help Strategies

Vaginal Moisturisers and Lubricants: A quick and effective way to combat dryness is by using vaginal moisturisers and lubricants, which can alleviate discomfort and enhance sexual satisfaction.

Local Oestrogen Therapy: For more persistent symptoms, a healthcare provider might suggest local oestrogen therapy. This treatment comes in various forms including vaginal creams, tablets, or rings, and can effectively restore tissue health.

Regular Sexual Activity: Maintaining regular sexual activity, either with a partner or through self-stimulation, can promote blood flow to the vaginal area, helping maintain its health and elasticity.

Pelvic Floor Exercises: Engaging in pelvic floor exercises can enhance vaginal tone and health. It's akin to giving your vaginal muscles a good workout to keep them sprightly and robust!

Hydration and Diet: Keeping the body hydrated and incorporating a diet rich in phytoestrogens (found in foods like soy, flaxseeds, and tofu) can provide some relief from symptoms. See chapter 27 for more on this.

Consult a Medical Provider: It is of paramount importance to consult with a healthcare provider to explore suitable treatments and therapies based on individual health profiles.

It's essential to step into this phase with knowledge and a readiness to embrace the changes while seeking avenues to enhance comfort and well-being. Vaginal dryness and atrophy, while common, does not have to be endured in silence.

Decreased Libido: When Your Desire Puts the Pause in Perimenopause

Feeling less 'in the mood' than usual? You're not alone. While there aren't exact statistics focusing specifically on libido decline during perimenopause, studies indicate that about 32-47% of women experience sexual dysfunction, which includes low libido, during their lifetime. A decline in libido is often a complex interplay of emotional, psychological, and biological factors. Stress, self-esteem, and emotional well-being can significantly contribute to your sexual desire, making it essential to look at your emotional health holistically.

Oestrogen doesn't just play a role in reproductive health; it's also pivotal in how you experience arousal and pleasure. When your oestrogen levels decline during perimenopause, it's not uncommon for your libido to wane as well.

Testosterone is also linked to libido and sexual satisfaction. During the perimenopause, testosterone levels can also decline, further contributing to a decreased sex drive. According to the *Journal of Women's Health*, a certain percentage of women have found relief from low libido through testosterone therapy, although it's not universally recommended due to lack of comprehensive research on long-term effects. Still, it's another piece of the intricate puzzle that is your sexual well-being during perimenopause. If you're considering hormone therapy, it may be worth discussing your testosterone levels along with oestrogen and progesterone with your healthcare provider (although not available on the NHS). See more on this in chapter 25.

One of the most effective ways to address a dip in sexual desire is open and honest dialogue with your partner. Whether it's discussing your fears, wishes, or even sexual fantasies, communication can strengthen your emotional connection, potentially reigniting your physical one. See chapter 17 on relationships for more information.

This phase of your life could be a golden opportunity to rekindle your sexual flame in new, exciting ways. Whether it's adopting more comfortable positions, experimenting with different forms of touch, or even introducing toys into the equation, stepping out of your comfort zone could inject new energy into your intimate life.

It might sound superficial, but a change in environment can significantly impact your mood and libido. Whether it's a weekend getaway, a candle-lit dinner at home, or even a bedroom makeover, think of these as 'reset buttons' for your sexual energy.

If your libido has persistently dipped and it's affecting your quality of life, consulting a healthcare provider or a certified sex therapist may be beneficial. Treatments could include hormone replacement therapy, or even specific libido-boosting medications like flibanserin, which has been shown to improve sexual desire in some studies.

Don't underestimate the power of self-love and self-care routines. Activities like mindfulness, relaxation techniques, or even taking a well-deserved break can help you understand your body better and could play a crucial role in regaining your sexual vitality.

Take a look at *"The UncompliKated Perimenopause Workbook"* for some great advice, exercises and tracking tools on self-love and self-care.

Self-Help Strategies

Maca Root: Known for its potential ability to boost libido, this root vegetable has been used traditionally to enhance fertility and sex drive.

Ginseng: This ancient root is touted for its ability to improve sexual function and has shown promise in several studies.

Fenugreek: While more commonly used to improve men's libido, some studies suggest that it can also help women.

Yoga: Practices focused on pelvic floor strengthening, like certain yoga poses, can sometimes aid in improving sexual health.

Perimenopause is not just about physiological changes; it's also an opportunity to rediscover yourself, your body, and your sexuality. A proactive approach to managing symptoms, open communication with your partner, and a dash of self-love can go a long way in helping you navigate this new chapter in your life's story of intimacy and self-discovery.

CHAPTER 15

The Ebb and Flow Reimagined

Navigating your new normal in menstrual cycles

As you might have already guessed, the perimenopause journey entails a smörgåsbord of changes to your menstrual cycle that we navigate through – the ups and downs, the heavy and the light, the early and the late arrivals of our menstrual cycles.

First and foremost, throw predictability out of the window. The only sure thing to do with your perimenopausal periods is that there is no sure thing. Genuinely. Some women have longer, some shorter, some heavier, some lighter, etc. so the only rule is that there is no rule.

Oh, the unpredictability that comes with perimenopause! It's like hosting a party where guests arrive fashionably late or sometimes a tad too early. The frequency of these irregular arrivals escalates as one approaches the golden age of 50. Remember, it's perfectly normal to have a few surprises along the way. Think of it as your body keeping you on your toes, adding a touch of spontaneity to life!

As you navigate through perimenopause, you might notice a fluctuation in the length of your menstrual cycles. It's a time of change and adaptation, where your body is fine-tuning itself to a new rhythm. A study indicates that about 92% of women experience these changes, marking a significant milestone in their journey to menopause.

You might notice that your menstrual cycle prefers a leisurely pace, extending its stay slightly. The menstrual cycle can lengthen by a couple of days or even more. You are not alone in this; almost 60% of women in their 40s experience a gradual increase in their menstrual cycle length.

Just when you thought you.ve seen it all, your menstrual cycle might throw a curveball, shortening its duration and arriving a tad sooner than expected. It's a swift, yet intense visit, reminding you to seize the day and live life with zest and zeal.

And the ebb and flow of your menstrual cycle might fluctuate too, sometimes resembling a gentle stream and at other times a robust river. These fluctuations are courtesy of the fluctuating levels of oestrogen and progesterone in your body.

Approximately 25% of women experience heavy periods during perimenopause, a phenomenon scientifically termed as menorrhagia. While it might seem like a grand gesture, don't hesitate to consult with your healthcare provider if things get too grandiose!

On the flip side, your period might choose a minimalist approach, gracing you with a light and breezy visit. This is a time to embrace the lighter side of life, perhaps indulging in activities that were otherwise put on hold. It's a gentle reminder that sometimes, less is indeed more.

Spotting in between periods can be akin to an unexpected guest popping by for a quick hello. This can be due to the delicate dance between oestrogen and progesterone, sometimes causing a little sprinkle of spotting between the main events. While it's a natural occurrence, it's not always convenient. Keeping a few panty liners in your bag, or maybe wearing period knickers (ones that are designed for periods and/or leaking are a great shout for perimenopause as they can provide a bit more 'security' and you can get bamboo ones too which help with thermo-regulating too).

Oh, the cramps! Sometimes, your body decides to throw a little tantrum, resulting in increased cramps during this time. It's your body's dynamic way of expressing itself, perhaps calling for a little extra TLC and pampering during these times. So, indulge in some self-care – you absolutely deserve it!

As we tread this path, you might find that PMS decides to turn up the volume a notch. But fear not, for you are equipped with resilience and grace to face this head-on. About 30-40% of women report a spike in PMS symptoms during perimenopause. Remember, a little bit of chocolate and a lot of self-love go a long way during these times.

Sometimes, your body might give you a sneak preview of the PMS gala, presenting PMS-like symptoms even when the grand event is yet to arrive. It's like a dress rehearsal, preparing you for the main show.

Self-Help Strategies

Track Your Cycle: The first step is to track your menstrual cycle. There are several apps available that can help you do this, allowing you to anticipate when you might need extra self-care, or you can use *The UncompliKated Perimenopause Journal* if you're a bit more old-school like I am. Pen and paper all the way for me!

Nutrition Matters: Foods rich in omega-3 fatty acids like salmon, or those full of antioxidants like berries, can help with hormonal balance. Nutritionists often recommend a balanced diet rich in fruits, vegetables, and lean proteins to ease symptoms.

Regular Exercise: Consistent exercise is beneficial for overall hormonal balance and can alleviate symptoms like bloating and mood swings. According to a study from *Obstetrics & Gynaecology*, regular exercise can also help manage irregular periods.

Stay Hydrated: Water is essential for every bodily function, including the regulation of menstrual cycles. Drinking enough water can help alleviate bloating and can also replace lost fluids during particularly heavy cycles.

Heat Therapy: Warm compresses or hot water baths can relieve muscle tension and alleviate menstrual cramps. Even a simple hot water bottle can do wonders. You can now buy fabulous longer hot water bottles now that stretch across your whole tummy that really make a difference.

Limit Sugar and Caffeine: (Sorry!) Excess sugar and caffeine can worsen hormonal imbalances, according to a study in the *American Journal of Clinical Nutrition*. Aim to cut back, especially during the luteal phase (the second half) of your cycle.

Natural Supplements: Herbal remedies like black cohosh, chasteberry, and evening primrose oil have been traditionally used for hormonal balance. However, always consult a healthcare provider before starting any new supplement. See the back of this book for more information on supplements.

Yoga and Meditation: Stress can aggravate hormonal imbalances. Practices like yoga and mindfulness meditation can help you stay centred and might even make your menstrual cycle more regular.

Over-the-Counter Remedies: Non-prescription NSAIDs like ibuprofen can help manage pain associated with menstrual cramps. But use these sparingly and consult your GP for long-term use.

Consult Your Health Care Provider: If menstrual irregularities become bothersome or if you have heavy bleeding, it might be time to consult a gynaecologist. They can offer treatments like hormonal birth control to regulate the menstrual cycle.

Bio-identical Hormones: These are structurally identical to the hormones produced by the body and can be prescribed to alleviate symptoms. Again, this requires consultation with a healthcare provider. (See more on the chapter on HRT.)

Acupuncture: Some studies, like one published in *Obstetrics & Gynaecology*, suggest that acupuncture can help regulate menstrual cycles and alleviate perimenopausal symptoms.

Mindfulness and Deep Breathing: These techniques not only reduce stress but can also help you deal with pain and emotional fluctuations more effectively.

Get Enough Sleep: Lack of sleep can exacerbate hormonal imbalances, so aim for seven to nine hours of quality sleep a night.

Speak to Others: Sometimes, just knowing you're not alone can make all the difference. Online forums, support groups, or simply talking to friends who are going through the same thing can provide valuable emotional support.

By adopting some of these strategies, you may find it easier to manage the ups and downs of menstrual cycle changes during perimenopause. And always remember, you're not alone on this journey. You are more than welcome to join my free support group on Facebook, Perimenopause with Kate Grosvenor, and then you've got a whole community behind you, sweetheart.

CHAPTER 16

Mental Health Matters

A compassionate look at the perimenopausal roller coaster

Perimenopause is often described as a hormonal roller coaster, but let's be honest, it's more like a theme park with a variety of rides – some thrilling, some downright terrifying. While much attention is given to the physical symptoms like hot flushes and night sweats, the impact on mental health is often swept under the rug.

But as the great Virginia Woolf said,

"One cannot think well, love well, sleep well, if one has not dined well."

And by "dining well," we mean addressing the full spectrum of perimenopausal symptoms, including the emotional and psychological ones.

Anxiety: The Unwanted Companion

The numbers speak for themselves on this one, and anxiety is much more common than you'd think! Anxiety doesn't discriminate, but statistics show that perimenopausal women are particularly susceptible. A study from the University of Cambridge indicated that 22% of women between 45-54 years old experience anxiety. In the UK alone, that means approximately 1.5 million women are dealing with this issue. Compared to the general population's anxiety prevalence of around 15%, it's evident that perimenopausal women face a higher risk.

The Causes (It's Not 'All in Your Head')

Hormonal Fluctuations: During perimenopause, the hormonal roller coaster isn't just affecting your physical body; it's also messing with your neurotransmitters. Changes in oestrogen and progesterone levels can result in heightened anxiety.

Life Changes: At this stage of life, many women are navigating significant transitions. Whether it's the kids flying the nest, shifts in career, or even changes in relationship dynamics, these life alterations can contribute to anxiety.

Self-Help Strategies

Mindfulness and Relaxation Techniques: Simple mindfulness exercises like deep breathing, progressive muscle relaxation, and guided visualisation can help you get a grip on your anxiety. According to the American Psychological Association, mindfulness-based stress reduction techniques have been effective in reducing anxiety symptoms.

Physical Exercise: Never underestimate the power of a good walk or a quick jog. Just thirty minutes of moderate exercise can release endorphins, your body's natural mood lifter. Studies have shown that exercise can be as effective as medication for treating mild to moderate anxiety and depression.

Social Support: Sometimes, talking it out with trusted friends and family can provide emotional relief and practical solutions. Don't underestimate the value of a good heart-to-heart.

Cognitive Behavioural Therapy (CBT): This form of psychotherapy has proven to be effective in treating anxiety disorders. It helps you become aware of negative thought patterns and equips you with strategies to combat them. There are some great exercises in *'The UncompliKated Perimenopause Workbook'* that I highly recommend.

Chamomile: Known for its calming effects, chamomile tea might help you feel more relaxed.

Lavender: Whether it's in the form of essential oils, teas, or bath salts, lavender has been shown to reduce symptoms of anxiety in some studies.

Passionflower: Used traditionally to treat anxiety and insomnia, this natural remedy has shown promise in small, early studies.

Omega-3 Fatty Acids: Found in foods like fish and flaxseed, omega-3s have anti-inflammatory properties that may help alleviate anxiety. (See the information on supplements at the back of this book).

Magnesium: Low magnesium levels have been linked to higher levels of anxiety. Supplements or a diet rich in magnesium (think leafy greens and nuts) could be beneficial.

Depression

Depression during perimenopause is not a fringe issue – it's a pressing concern that affects a large portion of women. According to the NHS, one in four women in the UK will require treatment for depression at some point in their lives. Moreover, women in their 40s and 50s form the largest demographic group using antidepressants in the country. Statistics indicate that up to 25% of perimenopausal women may experience depressive symptoms severe enough to seek medical treatment. Clearly, it's an issue that demands attention and understanding.

The Causes
Hormonal Changes: The hormonal flux that comes with perimenopause has more than just physical repercussions. Hormones like oestrogen can impact neurotransmitters like serotonin, which plays a significant role in mood regulation.

Physical Symptoms: Don't underestimate how much a poor night's sleep can affect your emotional well-being. Physical symptoms like night sweats that disturb your rest can have a cascading impact on your mood.

Self-Help Strategies
Talking Therapy: Whether it's with a qualified life coach, therapist or a trusted confidant, talking about your feelings and experiences can help. Cognitive behavioural therapy (CBT), a proven effective treatment for depression, can equip you with the tools you need to cope better with life's challenges.

Physical Exercise: It's not a cure-all, but regular exercise can stimulate endorphin release, which may help elevate your mood. Even a twenty-minute walk a few times a week can make a difference, as multiple studies have corroborated the benefits of exercise for mental health.

Mindfulness Meditation: Focusing on the present moment through mindfulness can help reduce symptoms of depression, according to a study published in the journal *JAMA Internal Medicine*.

Medication: Antidepressants like SSRIs (selective serotonin reuptake inhibitors) can offer relief for some, but it's vital to consult your healthcare provider for a diagnosis and treatment plan tailored for you.

St John's Wort: This plant has been used for ages to treat depression, though it's essential to consult your healthcare provider before starting any herbal treatments, especially if you are already on medication.

Omega-3 Fatty Acids: Some studies suggest that omega-3 supplements could have a mild antidepressant effect.

Vitamin D: Low levels of vitamin D have been associated with depression. Consider getting your levels checked and supplementing as necessary.

Folate-Rich Foods: Leafy greens and legumes contain folate, a B vitamin that has been linked to mood regulation.

Always consult a medical practioner before starting any supplements, especially if you have any pre-existing medical conditions.

Feeling Dead Inside: Emotional Numbness

We need to break the silence on this issue, and I'm here to speak out about the generally unspoken reality. Feeling emotionally numb is one of the less discussed but deeply unsettling experiences during perimenopause. While it's difficult to pinpoint exact statistics, the general consensus among healthcare providers is that emotional numbness is an underreported issue that affects a significant number of women. It's like watching your life unfold on a screen but not being able to engage with the plot or characters. When this emotional detachment sets in, even life's most joyful moments can feel dull and distant.

The Causes

Chronic Stress: The physical symptoms of perimenopause – hot flashes, insomnia, and weight gain, among others – can accumulate into chronic stress, further dulling your emotional responses.

Isolation: During perimenopause, the feeling of being misunderstood or 'different' can compound feelings of detachment, making you want to withdraw from even your closest relationships.

Self-Help Strategies

Social Support: It's essential to lean on your support network during this time. Friends and family who've been through similar experiences can provide invaluable emotional scaffolding. Remember, sometimes you need a village to get you through the tough times.

Mindfulness and Grounding Techniques: Learning mindfulness techniques like deep breathing and grounding exercises can help reconnect you with the present moment, providing an emotional 'anchor' when you feel adrift.

Physical Activity: Exercise is not just good for your body; it can also be a mood lifter. The endorphins released during exercise can help counteract feelings of emotional numbness.

Professional Help: Don't underestimate the value of a skilled coach or counsellor. They can offer targeted strategies to help you navigate your way out of the emotional fog and reconnect with your feelings.

Lavender Oil: Known for its calming properties, a few drops of lavender oil on your pillow or in a diffuser can help reduce stress, which could potentially ease feelings of numbness.

Valerian Root: This natural remedy is often used for sleep disorders and anxiety. Consult your healthcare provider before taking any herbal supplements, especially if you're already on medication.

Chamomile Tea: A warm cup of chamomile tea can have a calming effect, serving as a ritualistic moment of 'me-time' that might help you reconnect with yourself.

B Vitamins: A lack of B vitamins, particularly B12, has been associated with mood disorders. Consider incorporating more B-rich foods into your diet, like leafy greens and whole grains.

If you're experiencing emotional numbness during perimenopause, know that you're not alone and that it's okay to seek help. Emotional numbness may be one of the lesser-discussed symptoms of this life stage, but it's no less real or significant. So, don't hesitate to reach out for the support and treatment you deserve, because this too shall pass, and you're stronger than you think.

Also see the next chapter on relationships.

Panic Attacks/Disorder: The Emotional Tsunamis

The perimenopausal phase can sometimes be a perfect storm for triggering panic attacks. According to Mind, the mental health charity, around 5% of the UK population experiences panic attacks. However, research shows that perimenopausal women are at a higher risk, with rates doubling to about 10% among this group. That's a pretty significant leap, highlighting the need for more focused conversations and solutions around this topic.

The Causes

Hormonal Fluctuations: You guessed it! Those unpredictable hormones are back, causing an imbalance in neurotransmitters that can trigger panic attacks.

Increased Anxiety: Pre-existing anxiety can escalate during perimenopause, sometimes tipping over into full-blown panic attacks.

Self-Help Strategies

Breathing Techniques: One of the most effective tools you have is your breath. The 4-7-8 technique (breathe in for four seconds, hold for seven seconds, and exhale for eight seconds) has shown promise in calming the nervous system quickly.

Grounding Techniques: When you feel a panic attack coming on, ground yourself by focusing on your senses. Name five things you can see, four you can touch, three you can hear, two you can smell, and one you can taste. This can divert your mind and may help you ride out the panic wave.

Cognitive Behavioural Therapy (CBT): This is a longer-term strategy but incredibly effective for treating panic disorders. CBT helps you understand the patterns and thought processes that lead to panic attacks.

Regular Exercise: Aerobic exercise can often help in regulating the neurotransmitters that contribute to panic attacks, giving you a more natural defence against them.

Chamomile: Known for its calming properties, chamomile tea or supplements could be a natural way to lessen anxiety, thereby reducing the frequency of panic attacks.

Valerian Root: Much like it helps with anxiety and insomnia, valerian root can also be effective in reducing panic attacks. Consult your healthcare provider before starting any natural remedies, especially if you're already taking other medications. One of my favourite herbal teas called 'Calm' contains this root, and I've listed the Tea Pigs website in the resources section at the back of this book.

Passionflower: Studies have shown that passionflower can be as effective as some prescription medications for treating anxiety and panic disorders. Again, consult a healthcare provider before beginning a new supplement regimen.

Magnesium: A magnesium deficiency can contribute to increased anxiety. Taking magnesium supplements or eating magnesium-rich foods like leafy greens can help balance your mood. (See the supplements section for more information.)

Panic attacks during perimenopause are more common than many might think. While the experience can be terrifying, knowing the strategies to manage it can make all the difference. Remember, this is just another chapter in your journey. By equipping yourself with the right tools and knowledge, you'll be better prepared to navigate these emotional tsunamis. After all, even the roughest seas don't last forever.

Irritability: The Short Fuse

Irritability during perimenopause is so widespread that it's nearly a rite of passage. While comprehensive statistics are sparse, what we do know is compelling. According to a survey from the British Menopause Society, a staggering 90% of respondents reported mood changes, and irritability topped the charts. So, if you find yourself having a short fuse these days, take comfort in knowing you're far from alone – you're part of a rather large, albeit slightly irritable, sisterhood.

The Causes

Sleep Deprivation: It's not just babies and toddlers who get cranky without sleep; it affects grown-ups too. And let's face it, night sweats and insomnia are hardly conducive to a peaceful night's sleep.

Stress: Juggling symptoms like hot flushes, mood swings, and brain fog can naturally shorten anyone's emotional fuse. Add family and work responsibilities to the mix, and it's a recipe for irritability.   .

Self-Help Strategies

Time-Outs: Sometimes, the best thing you can do is remove yourself from the situation. Take a walk, step into another room, or simply close your eyes for a few minutes. This can help you gain a new perspective and re-join the world with a slightly longer fuse.

Physical Exercise: It can't be emphasised enough how beneficial exercise can be for mood regulation. A brisk thirty-minute walk, for instance, can release endorphins, helping to reset your emotional balance.

Deep Breathing: Practising deep-breathing techniques like the 4-7-8 method can help in immediate stress relief and may reduce irritability. I have a video on YouTube called 'Cocoa Breaths' that is another great breathing technique I created to help with irritability and anxiety.

Limit Stimulants: Caffeine and alcohol can exacerbate irritability. Try switching to herbal teas and non-alcoholic alternatives, especially later in the day.

Lavender: Known for its calming effects, lavender oil can be used in a diffuser or added to a warm bath.

Omega-3 Fatty Acids: Found in fish like salmon, omega-3s are known for their anti-inflammatory properties which can positively impact your mood.

St John's Wort: This natural remedy has been used for centuries to treat mood disorders. However, consult your healthcare provider before using St John's Wort as it can interfere with other medications.

Magnesium: As in the case of panic attacks, a magnesium deficiency can contribute to heightened stress and irritability. Consider a supplement after consulting with your healthcare provider. More information on supplements is available at the back of this book.

Irritability is a common but manageable symptom of perimenopause. With the right self-help strategies and perhaps a few natural remedies, it's entirely possible to lengthen that fuse and rediscover your equanimity. Remember, you're never alone on this journey. Feel empowered to talk about your experience; you'll likely find many women who are navigating the same irritable waters. And as they say, a problem shared is a problem halved – or at least, made more manageable.

Mood Swings: The Emotional Pendulum of Perimenopause

Mood swings during perimenopause are so ubiquitous that they're often shrugged off as a cliché. Yet, according to a study in the journal *Menopause*, a whopping 70% of women experience mood swings during this transitional period. In other words, if you feel like you're on an emotional roller coaster, you've got plenty of company in that theme park. What's more, these aren't just minor ups and downs; they can be potent enough to impact your daily life and relationships, making them a serious issue that needs addressing.

The Causes

Hormonal Fluctuations: Oestrogen and progesterone aren't just about reproductive health; they're also key players in regulating your mood. When these hormones fluctuate, so does your emotional stability.

External Stressors: The world doesn't pause for perimenopause. Work stress, family dynamics, and societal pressures continue, adding fuel to the emotional fire.

Self-Help Strategies

Mindfulness: Techniques like mindfulness meditation can help you become more aware of your emotional state. This self-awareness can be the first step in managing your mood swings more effectively.

Talking Therapy: Counselling or talking therapies such as CBT (cognitive behavioural therapy) offer a structured way to identify thought patterns and beliefs that might be contributing to your mood swings.

Regular Exercise: Physical activity releases endorphins, which can act as a natural mood stabiliser. Even a quick twenty-minute walk could make a world of difference. Remember, your *motion* creates your *emotion*.

Journaling: Keeping a mood diary can help you identify triggers and patterns. You'd be surprised how cathartic putting pen to paper can be. See *The UncompliKated Perimenopause Journal* for more ideas around this.

Chamomile Tea: Known for its calming effects, a cup of chamomile tea can offer a momentary respite from emotional chaos.

Vitamin B Complex: These vitamins are known to improve mood and are especially useful during periods of emotional stress.

Omega-3 Fatty Acids: As with irritability, omega-3s have mood-stabilising properties and can be found in fatty fish like salmon or in supplement form.

Acupuncture: Some women find relief from mood swings through acupuncture, although it's best to consult with a healthcare provider for a tailored treatment plan.

Mood swings might be a common side effect of perimenopause, but that doesn't mean you have to suffer in silence. With a range of self-help solutions and natural remedies available, you can seize control of your emotional pendulum and find a more balanced middle ground. The importance of mental well-being during this stage can't be overstated; after all, emotional health is just as vital as physical health, perhaps even more so in a stage of life filled with so much change

CHAPTER 17

Love in the Time of Hormones

Bridging the emotional moat in your relationships

I feel like this chapter should, in many ways, be called 'The Emotional Island.' Many women report feeling emotionally distant from their partners during perimenopause. It's as if an invisible wall has been erected between you and your loved ones. Conversations that used to flow easily now feel forced. Shared laughter that used to be a staple of your relationship now seems rare. It's not that the love has diminished, but the emotional bandwidth to engage at the same level as before seems to have shrunk. This emotional island can be a lonely place, even when surrounded by people who care about you.

The feelings of isolation and emotional distance during perimenopause are paradoxically both isolating and widely shared. Here, I expand on different types of relationships that might be affected, offering further strategies, statistics, and natural remedies.

The Causes

Irritability: According to the British Menopause Society, over 90% of women report mood changes during perimenopause, irritability being a leading concern.

Decreased Libido: Studies suggest that a large number of women experience a decline in libido during perimenopause, impacting emotional closeness.

See also the previous chapter on mindset and mental health.

Partners/Husbands – Building Bridges over Emotional Moats

Feeling emotionally distant during perimenopause can make a woman feel like she's become the guardian of her own emotional castle – complete with moats and a drawbridge that's very hesitant to lower. As we know from the *Journal of Women's Health*, this sensation is far from unique: a staggering 55% of women report feeling this way. So, let's explore how to repair those drawbridges and foster better connections with our partners or husbands.

First, let's revisit that statistic: 55% of women report feeling emotionally disconnected from their partners during this phase. To put that into context, if perimenopause were a game show, you'd have better odds of spinning the 'emotional distance' prize than you would of landing on 'sailing through unscathed.' And for couples already enduring life changes, that 55% figure can feel a bit like you've been thrown in the deep end – except no one's told you how to swim.

Self-Help Strategies

Open Communication: This strategy can't be overstated. The idea is to cut through the emotional fog with the bright light of clear dialogue. A 2019 study published in the journal *Family Process* found that couples who communicate effectively are ten times more likely to report a happy relationship than those who don't. When words fail, try the 'speaking without speaking' approach – a hug, a touch or even a knowing look can convey volumes.

Couples Therapy: If 55% of women are feeling emotionally distant, then it's likely that a fair number of couples are finding themselves in the therapist's office. And that's okay. According to the American Psychological Association, 75% of couples who opt for couples therapy find improvement in their relationships. So, the odds are in your favour, and keep the faith.

Scheduled Intimacy: At first glance, scheduling intimacy might sound as romantic as a tax audit. But relationship experts have found it can bring back the excitement and anticipation that spontaneity once offered. Think of it as a date night with benefits. The anticipation of knowing it's 'on the cards' can create a sense of excitement and closeness leading up to the moment.

Stay Active Together: According to the British Heart Foundation, just 150 minutes of moderate exercise a week can boost your mental well-being. Grab your partner and get moving, whether it's a dance class, a jog, or a YouTube workout video. Exercise releases endorphins, those magical chemicals that act as natural mood lifters.

Omega-3: I mentioned fish as a source, but for the piscatorially-averse, flaxseeds and walnuts are great alternatives. Omega-3 has been shown to improve mood and contribute to overall emotional well-being.

Vitamin D: Often known as the 'sunshine vitamin,' a lack of vitamin D can affect your mood. So, absorb that sunshine during walks or consider supplements.

Herbal Teas: Certain herbal teas like chamomile and valerian root are renowned for their calming properties, making them an excellent prelude to meaningful conversations or intimacy.

Maca Root: Used for centuries in traditional medicine, maca root is believed to boost libido. Though scientific evidence is still limited, some swear by its efficacy. As always, consult your healthcare provider before trying new supplements.

There is a dedicated section on supplements at the back of this book.

Feeling like an emotional island isn't on anyone's wish list for this life stage, but it's a common experience. Luckily, it doesn't have to be a life sentence. With targeted strategies like open communication, couples therapy, and scheduled intimacy, plus the support of natural remedies, you and your partner can rebuild that emotional bridge. And remember, even the most secure castles lower their drawbridges every now and then.

Children – More Than Just the Mum Hat

When you're navigating the roller coaster of perimenopause, the last thing you need is a teenager in the house going through their own hormonal circus. It's like mixing fire and petrol, expecting a rainbow. However, before we all start investing in flame-retardant clothing, let's take a breather and explore how to navigate this challenging but utterly normal life phase.

Research indeed confirms what you probably knew deep down – mums' moods impact the kids. According to a study published in *Developmental Psychology*, children are more likely to display behavioural problems if their mothers are experiencing mood swings or emotional issues. Just think about it: if mum's irritable, the house becomes a walking-on-egg-shells event, not unlike the finals of the *Great British Bake Off*.

When it comes to teenagers, a study by the *Journal of Adolescence* reveals that teens are sensitive to parents' mood fluctuations – even if they pretend they've got earphones super-glued permanently to their ears. So, the stakes are high, especially if you're dealing with both perimenopause and teenage turbulence.

Self-Help Strategies : For Mums

Quality Time: You might feel like you're being pulled in a million directions, what with hot flushes and mood swings. Nevertheless, research from the *Journal of Marriage and Family* shows that it's quality over quantity that counts when spending time with your children. So, even if you can manage just twenty minutes of undistracted conversation, make it count.

Open Discussions: Studies have indicated that a parent's openness can foster emotional intelligence in children. If mum can talk about her feelings in a candid yet age-appropriate way, kids are more likely to open up too. This doesn't mean laying all your emotional cards on the table; think of it more as showing them a few from your hand.

Self-Help Strategies : For Kids

Active Listening: Teach your children the art of active listening. This equips them to better understand you and vice versa. The American Academy of Paediatrics recommends active listening as a way to improve parent-child communication.

Expressive Arts: Encourage your child to express their feelings through art, writing or music. Expressive arts can act as emotional outlets and improve mental well-being.

Self-Help Strategies: For the Family

Lavender Oil: A dab of lavender oil on your pillow or a few drops in a diffuser can help ease stress and improve sleep for everyone in the household. Lavender has been proven to reduce cortisol, the stress hormone.

Valerian Root Tea: Known for its calming properties, valerian root can be an excellent pre-bedtime ritual for both you and your teenager. Just make sure to check for any possible side effects or interactions with other medications you may be taking.

Family Yoga: *The British Journal of Sports Medicine* suggests that yoga can reduce stress and improve mental well-being. Turn it into a family activity to boost everyone's spirits and enhance bonding.

Juggling perimenopause and motherhood – especially with teenagers in the mix – is no small feat. However, quality time and open discussions can act like the safety nets in this emotional high-wire act. Add in some natural remedies to your routine, and you might just make it through with everyone still speaking to each other.

Remember, you're not just wearing the mum hat; you're wearing the human hat too. Give yourself the grace to experience your emotions and the wisdom to manage them constructively. After all, families are like tapestries – each thread, no matter how tangled, contributes to a beautiful whole.

Friends – Your Lifelines: More Than Just a Cuppa and a Chat

Let's be honest, when you're going through perimenopause, sometimes your friends can feel like your personal superheroes. They can't fly or shoot webs from their wrists, but they're uncanny at knowing when to drop a hilarious meme into your inbox or showing up with a bottle of wine right when you need it. But the benefits of friendship aren't just a subjective feel-good factor; there's actual science behind it, proving that friendship is good for your health – especially during times like perimenopause.

Brace yourself for this statistic: according to a meta-analysis published in the journal *PLOS Medicine*, strong social bonds can increase your lifespan by up to 50%. Yes, you read that right, a whopping 50%! It turns out that friendship is more effective than most medicines in the cabinet. Also, according to the World Health Organisation, people with strong social connections are generally happier, less stressed, and, quite frankly, they get fewer colds. So, perhaps ditching that cold medicine for a night out with friends might not be such a bad idea after all!

But let me be candid: perimenopause can put a bit of a strain on friendships. When you're struggling with mood swings and irritability, the idea of socialising can sometimes seem as appealing as nails on a chalkboard. However, this is when you need your friends the most. Isolation and loneliness can exacerbate perimenopausal symptoms, according to the British Menopause Society. So, keep those friendships burning, even if it's just a quick text or a ten-minute phone call to vent about the fact that your internal thermostat seems to be stuck on 'tropical jungle'.

Self-Help Strategies

Regular Check-ins: The frequency of social interactions correlates positively with emotional well-being. This doesn't mean you need to organise a weekend retreat with your mates (although that would be fun). Sometimes just a quick WhatsApp message to ask how they're doing can make all the difference – for both of you.

Honest Conversations: I absolutely hate the 'F' word...'fine'. Transparency and vulnerability can be therapeutic. Openness in friendships is shown to reduce feelings of loneliness and isolation. So, don't hesitate to say, "I'm feeling a bit off today," instead of the automatic, "I'm fine." You'd be surprised how liberating honesty can be.

Group Activities: Find a group activity that you and your friends can enjoy together. It could be anything from a book club to a cooking class. The social interaction will lift your spirits, and group activities offer a great distraction from any pesky symptoms you might be experiencing.

Walk in Nature: There's more to a walk than just stretching your legs. A walk in nature with a friend can elevate your mood, and it's backed by science. According to a study in Environmental Science & Technology, spending time in nature can reduce stress and improve mental well-being. Plus, you get a good boost of vitamin D – just don't forget the sunscreen!

Herbal Teas: When you catch up for your customary coffee, maybe switch to herbal teas like chamomile or peppermint, which are known for their calming effects. Chamomile tea is said to help alleviate symptoms of anxiety.

Essential Oils: Some essential oils are known to improve mood. Take a small vial of lavender or citrus essential oil when you meet your friends. A quick sniff can help reduce stress and elevate mood, according to the Journal of Alternative and Complementary Medicine.

There's an old saying, "Friendship isn't a big thing, it's a million little things.". This couldn't be more accurate, especially during the emotional turbulence of perimenopause. From that reassuring text message to the empathetic ear, your friends are your lifelines. So, keep the communication channels open, enjoy shared activities, and consider incorporating some natural mood-boosters into your social activities. After all, with friends like these, who needs super-heroes?

Parents – The Dual Role: Between a Rock and an Older Place

Ah, parents. They've seen us through our terrible twos, our awkward teenage years, and now, as we venture into the realm of perimenopause, the tables are somewhat turning. Many women find themselves part of the 'sandwich generation', caring for both their children and their ageing parents. According to the Pew Research Centre, one in three adults in their 40s and 50s is part of this unique demographic. If you're in this boat, chances are you're not only juggling mood swings and hot flushes but also parent-teacher meetings and medical appointments for Mum or Dad. It's no wonder you're feeling a bit frazzled.

Women in the sandwich generation, particularly those in perimenopause, experience higher levels of stress than other demographics. In fact, the stress levels are significantly higher than in men of the same age or women without these caregiving responsibilities. If you find yourself feeling overwhelmed, it's not your imagination – you're genuinely handling more stress than most.

The fluctuating hormones and stress of perimenopause can have a dual impact when you're caring for ageing parents. Irritability and fatigue can make us less patient, affecting the quality of care we can offer and straining the parent-child relationship further. We love our parents, but let's be honest, taking care of them while experiencing hormonal upheaval is like trying to assemble IKEA furniture – challenging and best not attempted alone.

It's worth mentioning that our emotional state during perimenopause can impact our parents as well. They may not fully understand the physiological changes you're going through and might misinterpret your irritability or emotional distance as a sign of neglect or waning affection. Remember, they have their own set of age-related concerns, and your emotional availability matters to them.

Self-Help Strategies

Share the Load: No one has ever won an award for 'Doing It All on Their Own While Making It Look Easy.' Studies indicate that sharing the caregiving burden among siblings or other family members can reduce both emotional and physical stress. Schedule a family meeting to discuss ways to share responsibilities. Even something as simple as having a sibling take over a doctor's appointment can be a big relief.

Professional Help: While family counselling may seem like a drastic step, it can be a saving grace. A therapist can mediate and provide coping mechanisms that can significantly reduce stress and familial tension. Counselling can improve communication in families significantly.

Mindfulness and Meditation: Yes, it's not just a buzzword. The practice of mindfulness can help lower stress levels. According to the *Journal of Behavioural Medicine*, mindfulness-based stress reduction programs have shown to reduce symptoms of stress in caregivers.

Natural Supplements: Stress-relief supplements like valerian root can help you manage stress without the side effects of medication. A study published in the journal BMC Complementary Medicine and Therapies found that valerian root could effectively reduce stress without impacting the ability to focus or execute tasks.

Nutrition: Eating foods rich in B-vitamins like whole grains and leafy greens can provide an additional layer of stress relief. Consider making a weekly meal plan that includes these stress-busting foods. As always, please consult a medical practioner, especially if you have any pre-existing medical conditions.

Being in the sandwich generation while going through perimenopause is a lot like being a juggler at a circus – except no one's clapping, and all the balls are on fire. But with some planning, professional guidance, and a sprinkle of natural remedies, you can make this challenging phase more manageable for everyone involved. And who knows? You might even get a standing ovation from your family for pulling it off.

Employers and Co-Workers – Work-Life Balance: Navigating the Hormonal High Seas of Office Politics

If the emotional roller coaster of perimenopause had a boardroom edition, it would probably involve navigating tricky relationships with employers and co-workers. Before you dive head-long into a spreadsheet or inadvertently snap at your boss, let's pause and take stock. According to a study by the British Menopause Society a staggering one in four women considered leaving their jobs due to the challenges posed by perimenopause symptoms. Now, that's a statistic that should make any HR department sit up and take notice.

When you're struggling with hot flushes, mood swings, and irritability, the last thing you want to do is negotiate with an employer or handle a co-worker's snarky comments. Emotional symptoms of perimenopause can strain professional relationships, leading to misunderstandings and making the workplace feel like a combat zone. It's like trying to solve a complex algebra equation while riding a unicycle – doable, but why make life harder than it has to be?

You're not the only one impacted by the symptoms you're experiencing; your boss and colleagues are also on the receiving end of your mood fluctuations. Whether it's a sharp reply in a meeting or visible disinterest during a presentation, your behaviour can set the tone for the entire team. A survey by the British Occupational Health Research Foundation found that 35% of women felt they were managed unfairly during their perimenopause transition, indicating that there's not only room for improvement but a crying need for it.

Self-Help Strategies

Transparency: While we're not advocating turning team meetings into therapy sessions, open dialogue with your employer can go a long way. Research published in the Harvard Business Review shows that transparency about your needs and challenges significantly improves job satisfaction and reduces stress. Don't be afraid to ask for flexible working hours or a more comfortable workspace.

Boundaries: Easier said than done, but setting clear work-life boundaries is crucial for emotional well-being. Maintaining distinct borders between your personal and professional life lowers stress and improves overall life satisfaction. If you can't leave work at the office, at least don't bring it into your emotional space.

Chamomile Tea: More than just a comforting warm drink, chamomile tea has anti-anxiety properties. A study published in the journal *Molecular Medicine Reports* found that chamomile could reduce symptoms of mild to moderate generalised anxiety disorder. Consider sipping some before a stressful meeting.

Lavender Oil: Sleep is a critical aspect of managing perimenopausal symptoms, and poor sleep can wreak havoc on your work performance.

Lavender oil can improve sleep quality. Maybe keep a small bottle in your office drawer for those times you need a calming influence.

Ashwagandha: This herb is a bit of a star player in the world of natural stress relief. A study published in the *Indian Journal of Psychological Medicine* found that ashwagandha

significantly reduces cortisol levels, the hormone responsible for stress. Incorporating this into your daily routine could make those office pressures more manageable.

If the office is starting to feel like a battleground and your keyboard like a weapon, it's time to take some proactive steps to safeguard your professional relationships during perimenopause. Open communication, boundaries, and a little natural help can keep you from boarding the 'Resignation Express.' After all, you've built your career through years of hard work; don't let perimenopause take that away from you. Cheers to reclaiming your work-life balance, one strategic move at a time.

In general, if perimenopause has you feeling like a castaway on an emotional island, remember you're far from alone. Armed with these expanded strategies and insights, may your voyage back to emotional closeness be swift and steady.

CHAPTER 18

Beauty and the Hormonal Best

Your evolving skin and hair story

In this journey of metamorphosis that we women traverse during perimenopause, our skin and hair don't want to be left behind in the transformation. As we voyage further, you might notice that your outer shell begins to showcase a vivid canvas of changes, a testament to the vibrant journey within.

Our skin often narrates the tales of time, and during perimenopause, and it seems to have a vivid storyline. As we sail through these changing tides, our skin may sometimes feel a tad dry, a bit itchy, and perhaps a touch less elastic, which is quite normal for nearly 50% of women experiencing perimenopause.

Formication, a rather fancy term for that peculiar sensation of tiny ants marching across your skin, might make an appearance during this time. The main culprit behind this is lower oestrogen levels. It's a quirky little interlude, where your nerves decide to play a friendly prank on you. Rest assured, this sensation, experienced by a considerable number of women, is just your body's way of keeping things interesting.

The moisture-rich skin you're accustomed to might play hide-and-seek during this phase. It's not uncommon to experience bouts of dry skin, a phenomenon noted by approximately 75% of women stepping into their glorious 50s. It's time to shower your skin with a little extra nourishment and moisture, as you would nurture a budding flower. See more in the chapter on skin care, which is of paramount importance at this time.

During this transitional phase, your skin might develop a slight itch for attention, quite literally. Itchy skin can be a gentle nudge from your body, inviting you to indulge in soothing skin rituals. Consider this a golden opportunity to pamper yourself with luxurious skin treatments that calm and soothe the itch away.

Oh, and the adolescent visitor might make a cameo during perimenopause. Acne, that once dreaded teenage guest, might pop up to say a little hello, thanks to the fluctuating hormone levels. But fret not, for you are now armed with the wisdom and grace to manage these surprise visits with aplomb.

You might also notice a gentle shift in your skin's palette, showcasing a rich tapestry of shades and hues. Skin discolouration is a natural part of the journey, a beautiful testament to the rich and varied experiences etched on your skin, akin to a beautiful painting evolving over time.

During this period, our skin decides to let go of its stringent adherence to elasticity, opting for a relaxed, laid-back approach. It might not spring back as eagerly as it once did, a gentle reminder to embrace the softness and grace that comes with time. After all, every fine artwork is characterised by soft curves and gentle lines, isn't it?

And just when you think you're more than itchy enough (thank you *very* much) your scalp decides to join in on the itch-fest too! It's an open invitation to indulge in soothing scalp massages, perhaps turning it into a weekly ritual of relaxation and pampering. Embrace this itchy interlude as a golden ticket to self-care and nourishment.

Every now and then, your face might decide to host a little blush party, presenting a radiant flush that lights up your countenance. It's like nature's way of adding a touch of rosy glow, keeping things vibrant and lively. Try and include soothing and calming products in your skin care routine.

Thinning hair is quite a common guest during this time, visiting about 40% of women in their perimenopausal stage and our hair might decide to take a slight retreat, shedding a little more than usual. Hair loss, experienced by a considerable percentage of women during this phase, is a gentle reminder to nurture and nourish your locks with loving care.

Your vibrant mane might also showcase a touch of fragility, opting for a softer, more brittle texture. It's an invitation to indulge in deep conditioning treatments, pampering your tresses with the love and care they deserve. Remember, even the finest silk requires gentle handling.

And while we're on the subject of hair, a touch of rugged charm might grace your facial canvas too, a few extra whiskers here or there, but nothing that a good pair of tweezers and a magnifying mirror can't fix. (But on a random side note, don't get a super-magnifying one as no woman needs that much close-up info!)

Our nails too might be a tad brittle. Indulge in nurturing nail care rituals. I keep a very hydrating hand cream on my bedside table for that last thing top up before bed.

Change is inevitable, and your skin, hair and nails, might not be the twenty-year-old version, but they can look and feel amazing, just with some beautiful care behind them. Think of the extra attention as self-loving rituals that are a way to show yourself how much you care.

Skin Care During Perimenopause: A Journey of Graceful Transformation

As you navigate through the perimenopausal period, skincare emerges as a sanctuary of self-care and rejuvenation. During this time, the skin undergoes several alterations, driven by hormonal fluctuations that can affect its texture, tone, and elasticity. According to a study in the *International Journal of Women's Dermatology,* over 50% of women experience noticeable changes in their skin texture and elasticity during this period.

Adopting a skincare ritual (I just prefer that word to 'routine' as it has more goddess-like qualities) that addresses these changes not only fosters healthier skin but also nurtures a deeper connection with yourself, transforming the skin care routine into a ritual of self-love and acceptance.

Understanding the nuances of these transformations and equipping yourself with knowledge can pave the way for a graceful journey through perimenopause. This chapter delves into the intricacies of skincare during perimenopause, offering guidance and tips to navigate this transitional phase with confidence and grace.

Skin Changes During Perimenopause

Perimenopause brings with it a host of skin changes, owing to the hormonal roller coaster that characterises this period. A gradual decrease in oestrogen levels influences several aspects of skin health, leading to noticeable shifts in skin texture, tone, and elasticity. Let's delve deeper into these changes, offering a comprehensive view of what happens to the skin during this time.

During perimenopause, the body witnesses a decline in the production of oestrogen, a hormone intrinsically linked to skin health. Oestrogen is known to promote production of collagen, a protein responsible for maintaining skin's elasticity and suppleness. As oestrogen levels dip, the skin starts to lose its youthful vigour, paving the way for various alterations including dryness, wrinkles, and loss of firmness. Moreover, changes in the levels of other hormones like progesterone and testosterone further contribute to changes in skin health, including increased oiliness or adult acne.

Understanding the hormonal dynamics of perimenopause can empower individuals to adapt their skin care routines, incorporating products and habits that cater to the evolving needs of the skin.

The gradual decrease in collagen and elastin production during perimenopause affects the skin's ability to retain moisture and maintain its firmness. This can lead to dryness, a pronounced appearance of fine lines, and a loss of skin's youthful bounce. Moreover, the reduction in natural oils exacerbates dryness, leaving the skin craving hydration and nourishment.

To counteract these changes, incorporating hydrating ingredients in your skin care routine can be a game-changer. Look for products enriched with hyaluronic acid, a moisture-binding ingredient that helps retain water in the skin, restoring its plumpness and vitality. Moreover, nourishing oils like rosehip oil, argan oil, and jojoba oil can replenish the skin's lipid barrier, offering a boost of moisture and nourishment.

As perimenopause progresses, you might notice an increase in wrinkles and fine lines. This happens due to the decline in collagen and elastin, the proteins responsible for skin's elasticity and firmness. According to Dr. Shirin Lakhani, an aesthetic doctor, "After the age of 30, we lose approximately 1% of our collagen each year, and this process accelerates during perimenopause."

To counteract these changes, consider adopting these measures:

Hyaluronic Acid Treatments

Hyaluronic acid can draw moisture into the skin, helping to smooth out fine lines temporarily.

Regular Facial Massages

Facial massages can help stimulate collagen production, enhancing skin's elasticity over time. Why not try a Gua Sha or facial roller? You can use these at home when you are massaging your face to boost circulation and stimulate collagen production. You could also consider periodic professional facial treatments that focus on lifting and firming the skin.

Hyperpigmentation and Age Spots

Hyperpigmentation and age spots often become more noticeable during perimenopause. Fluctuating hormones can lead to an increase in melanin production, which is the cause of these spots. Melasma, or hormonal pigmentation, is commonly triggered during perimenopause, and it's essential to address this concern with targeted treatments.

Several ingredients can help lighten hyperpigmentation and age spots. I suggest using products containing Vitamin C, liquorice extract, or kojic acid, all of which are known for their skin brightening properties. (Note: if you are using a Vitamin C serum or treatment, please make sure you apply an SPF daily as it can make your skin more sensitive to UV radiation.)

Chemical Peels

Chemical peels can be a game-changer in treating hyperpigmentation as they help in shedding the top layer of the skin, revealing a more even complexion underneath. You can try an at-home peel and start with milder at-home peels which contain AHAs or BHAs to gradually improve skin's texture and tone. For more pronounced hyperpigmentation, consider professional chemical peel treatments under the guidance of a dermatologist.

Changes in Skin Texture

During perimenopause, you may notice changes in your skin texture, including increased dryness and a decrease in firmness. Changes in oestrogen levels can lead to thinner skin and a loss of moisture, which can significantly affect skin's texture.

To address dryness, look for products that contain hydrating ingredients such as glycerine and hyaluronic acid.

Nutrition and Supplementation

Nutrition plays a pivotal role in skin health during perimenopause. A study published in the *American Journal of Clinical Nutrition* found that higher vitamin C intake was associated with less likelihood of a wrinkled appearance among middle-aged women.

Including omega fatty acids in your diet can help in maintaining skin's moisture levels and improving its texture.

Incorporate sources of omega fatty acids in your diet, such as flaxseeds, walnuts, and fatty fish to get the nutrients into your diet. Alternatively, or additionally, consider supplements such as fish oil or flaxseed oil to boost your omega fatty acid intake.

See more in the supplements section at the back of this book.

Skincare Products Recommended for Perimenopausal Skin
Gentle Cleansing

As the skin undergoes transformations during perimenopause, it requires a gentle touch, especially when it comes to cleansing. Opting for a mild, sulphate-free cleanser can prevent the skin from being stripped of its natural oils, maintaining its moisture barrier intact. Include cleansing balms or oils that dissolve impurities without disrupting the skin's natural pH balance. I recommend double cleansing, especially if you wear make-up. The first cleanse would be with a cleansing balm or oil, and the second with a creamy or hydrating cleanser.

Hydration and Moisturising

When navigating the perimenopausal period, hydration stands as a linchpin in maintaining the skin's vitality. The declining levels of oestrogen contribute to a diminished capacity of the skin to retain moisture, necessitating a focused approach to hydration.

Start with incorporating a rich moisturiser that contains ingredients known to bolster the skin's moisture barrier, such as ceramides and fatty acids. Products containing hyaluronic acid, a powerhouse hydrating agent, can also aid in replenishing the skin's water content, giving it a plump and youthful appearance. Don't forget the delicate neck and décolletage areas, which often show signs of aging more quickly and require dedicated care.

Furthermore, integrate a weekly hydrating mask into your regimen to provide a surge of moisture, addressing dryness and flakiness that often accompany this stage. A nightly ritual of applying a deeply nourishing cream can work wonders in rejuvenating the skin as you sleep.

Keeping your skin well-moisturised can help mitigate the common dryness experienced during perimenopause.

Sun Protection

Sun protection remains a critical component of skin care at every age, but gains even more significance during perimenopause. The skin becomes more susceptible to the harmful effects of UV radiation due to the thinning of the epidermis. Implement a broad-spectrum sunscreen with a high SPF into your daily routine, even on cloudy days or during the winter.

Consider products with added antioxidants like vitamin C to offer additional protection against environmental aggressors, including pollution and free radicals. Incorporate sun protection in your makeup products as well for an added layer of defence.

Targeted Treatments

The inclusion of targeted treatments in your skin care regimen can provide significant benefits during perimenopause.

Retinol

Retinol helps in rejuvenating the skin cells and promotes a more youthful skin texture and tone.

Niacinamide

Niacinamide works to protect your skin from environmental damages and also helps to calm the skin, so it's great to use in perimenopause.

Antioxidants

According to a report in the journal *Dermatologic Surgery*, topical antioxidants can provide skin protection against environmental damage and prevent signs of aging.

The Role of Exfoliation

Exfoliation aids in removing dead skin cells, fostering a radiant complexion. Incorporate gentle exfoliation into your skin care routine to promote healthy skin cell turnover, which tends to slow down during perimenopause.

Nutritional Support and Hydration

Navigating through perimenopause smoothly requires a holistic approach that goes beyond topical treatments. What you nourish your body with plays a vital role in determining the health and appearance of your skin.

Importance of Hydration

Hydration is not only about what you apply on the skin but also about what you ingest. Drinking sufficient amounts of water throughout the day can aid in maintaining the skin's elasticity and plumpness. Consider infusing your water with skin-loving ingredients such as cucumber or lemon to add a flavour twist and additional benefits.

Furthermore, hydrating teas with ingredients like chamomile, hibiscus or green tea can offer a soothing and skin-boosting alternative to regular beverages, aiding in maintaining a luminous complexion from the inside out.

Nutritional Supplements

As the nutrient absorption capacity might decline during perimenopause, supplementing your diet with vital nutrients can be beneficial. Supplements rich in omega-3 fatty acids, vitamin E, and collagen can aid in maintaining the skin's health. Always consult with a healthcare provider before introducing any new supplements to your routine.

Lifestyle Adjustments

To complement your skin care and nutrition regimen, adopting lifestyle habits that foster overall well-being is crucial during perimenopause.

Stress Management

Perimenopause can sometimes be a period of increased stress levels due to hormonal fluctuations. Managing stress effectively can prevent it from taking a toll on your skin. Incorporate practices such as meditation, yoga, and mindfulness into your daily routine to foster a sense of calm and balance.

Adequate Sleep

Quality sleep is vital for the regeneration of skin cells. Initiate a soothing bedtime ritual to encourage better sleep, which might include a warm bath, reading, or listening to calming music. Ensure you get at least seven to eight hours of sleep to allow your skin to repair and rejuvenate overnight.

Tailoring a Skin Care Regimen to Individual Needs

Navigating the perimenopausal phase involves embracing a period of profound change, not only hormonally but also in how your skin responds to these shifts. Just as every individual experiences perimenopause uniquely, the skin care regimen should be meticulously tailored to suit one's specific needs. The one-size-fits-all approach is outdated, particularly during a period as dynamic as perimenopause. Now, more than ever, personalised skin care is key. A good place to start is talking to your facialist about how they feel your skin is right now and ask what products they recommend. Also, be aware that you will probably have to swap your skincare with the seasons.

Hormone Replacement Therapy (HRT)

For some individuals, changes in skin condition during perimenopause might be significantly influenced by hormonal fluctuations. In such cases, specialists might recommend hormone replacement therapy (HRT) as a part of the skin care regimen. HRT can sometimes play a vital role in maintaining skin's vitality during perimenopause, by potentially mitigating the effects of hormonal fluctuations on the skin.

Laser Treatments

To tackle issues like hyperpigmentation, loss of elasticity, and fine lines, specialists might recommend laser treatments. Laser treatments can be an excellent option for those looking to address specific skin concerns like pigmentation or loss of firmness, offering targeted strategies.

Embarking on the perimenopausal journey with a skin care regimen that is finely attuned to your unique needs can be both empowering and rewarding. The journey through perimenopause is a passage to rediscovering yourself, and a personalised skin care regimen can be your trusted companion, aiding you in blossoming into a new phase of beauty and vitality.

Remember, consultation with a skin specialist or a dermatologist can provide a detailed insight into creating a skin care regimen that resonates perfectly with your skin's unique symphony during this time of transformation

CHAPTER 19

No Snooze, You Lose

Decoding sleepless nights, lack of umph, and running on fumes

Ah, sleep . . . That blissful state where we escape from the world and recharge our batteries. But what happens when sleep becomes as elusive as a unicorn? Welcome to the perimenopausal sleep saga, where counting sheep might just turn into counting hot flushes. In this chapter, we'll delve into the nitty-gritty of sleep disruptions, insomnia, and the resulting fatigue that many women experience during perimenopause. So, grab a cup of chamomile tea, and let's get started.

Sleep Disruptions – Insomnia

If you find yourself tossing and turning at night, staring at the ceiling as if it holds the answers to life's mysteries, you're not alone. My brain loves to ruminate over questions like "Do penguins have knees?" or "How does a man who drives a snow plough get to work in the morning?".

According to the NHS, up to 61% of perimenopausal women in the UK experience sleep disruptions. In the US, the numbers are similar, with 56% of perimenopausal women reporting sleep issues. That's more than half of women in this life stage, making it a significant concern that goes beyond mere inconvenience.

The statistics are eye-opening, aren't they? In the UK alone, that's potentially millions of women lying awake at night, contemplating everything from their to-do lists to the meaning of life. And let's not forget our sisters across the pond in the US, where the numbers are nearly as staggering. This isn't a minor issue; it's an insomnia epidemic that's affecting women on both sides of the Atlantic.

The fact that over half of perimenopausal women are experiencing sleep disruptions means that if you're going through this, you're in the majority. You're part of a large and not-so-restful sisterhood. So, if misery loves company, take solace in knowing that many are sharing in your nightly vigils.

To put it in perspective, if we consider that there are approximately 13 million women aged 45-64 in the UK, based on the NHS statistics, that would mean around 7.9 million women could be experiencing sleep disruptions. In the US, with an estimated 42 million women in the same age bracket, that's a whopping 23.5 million women potentially staring at their ceilings each night.

It's not just a one-off event either. Many women report that these sleep disruptions occur frequently, sometimes many times a week, adding up to a significant amount of lost sleep over time. This isn't just an occasional annoyance; it's a recurring issue that can have a profound impact on quality of life.

The repercussions of sleep disruptions go beyond just feeling tired. Lack of sleep can affect your mood, cognitive function, and even your physical health. Studies have shown that chronic sleep deprivation can lead to issues like increased stress, decreased immune function, and a higher risk of chronic conditions like heart disease and diabetes.

Self-Help Strategies

Sleep Hygiene: Creating a bedtime routine and sticking to it can help signal to your body that it's time to wind down. This could include activities like reading, taking a warm bath, or even some gentle stretching.

Limit Stimulants: Avoiding caffeine and alcohol close to bedtime can also make a significant difference. These substances can interfere with your sleep cycle and the quality of your sleep. Sugar before bed is also not a great idea as it might make your heart race in an effort to burn it off (see more on insulin resistance).

Brain Dumping: This is amazing before bed if you are the kind of woman whose brain is full of chatter at night time. Once you get everything off your head, it's easier to sleep, but also, if you wake up in the middle of the night thinking you've forgotten something you can tell your brain it's ok, you've written it down. You can do this just on plain paper or I have a brain journal that's great if you want to categorise and sort things. You can find it on my website (www.kategrosvenorbooks.com) or on Amazon.

Consult a Healthcare Provider: If sleep disruptions become a chronic issue, it may be time to consult a healthcare provider for a thorough evaluation and treatment options. This could include sleep studies, medication, or hormone replacement therapy as potential solutions.

By understanding the reality, prevalence, and impact of sleep disruptions, you can take steps to address this issue head-on. You're not alone in this, and help is available. With the right strategies, you can improve your sleep and, by extension, your overall well-being.

Disrupted Sleep

Disrupted sleep isn't just about having trouble falling asleep; it's also about waking up frequently during the night. According to a study by the British Menopause Society, a staggering 79% of perimenopausal women report waking up at least once during the night. That's nearly four out of every five women in this life stage. It's like a nightly game of musical beds, only you're the only player, and the music is your own internal hormonal symphony.

When we talk about 79% of perimenopausal women experiencing disrupted sleep, we're talking about a vast number of women. In the UK alone, that could equate to over 10 million women waking up in the middle of the night. In the US, the numbers would be even higher, potentially affecting over 33 million women. That's a lot of people not getting their beauty sleep!

If you're waking up in the middle of the night, you're in good company. With nearly eight out of ten women experiencing the same issue, you're far from alone. It's almost like a nightly club that no one wants to be a part of, but membership is automatic once you hit perimenopause.

If we break it down further, let's say the average woman wakes up once a night. Over a week, that's seven instances of disrupted sleep. Over a year, that's 365 instances. Over the course of perimenopause, which can last several years, we're talking about thousands of instances of disrupted sleep. That's not just a blip; that's a significant chunk of your life affected by poor sleep.

For some women, waking up once a night might even be a good night. Many report waking up multiple times, leading to fragmented sleep that's far from restorative. It's like trying to complete a puzzle with pieces constantly being removed and added back in; you never quite get the full picture.

The impact of disrupted sleep is far-reaching. It affects your mood, your cognitive abilities, and even your physical health. Studies have shown that disrupted sleep can lead to increased levels of stress hormones, decreased immune function, and a higher risk of developing chronic conditions like hypertension and diabetes.

Self-Help Strategies
Temperature Control: Night sweats are a common cause of waking up during the night. Consider using bamboo sheets and sleepwear which are thermoregulating, or even a cooling mattress pad, to help regulate your body temperature.

Mindfulness Techniques: Practices like deep breathing or progressive muscle relaxation can help you fall back asleep more quickly when you do wake up.

Consult a Healthcare Provider: If disrupted sleep becomes a chronic issue, it may be time to consult a healthcare provider for a thorough evaluation and treatment options. This could include medication, hormone replacement therapy (HRT), or even cognitive behavioural therapy for insomnia (CBT-I).

Understanding the scope and impact of disrupted sleep during perimenopause can empower you to take steps to improve your sleep quality. You're not alone in this struggle, and there are effective strategies and treatments available to help you get the rest you need.

Insomnia
Insomnia is the grandmaster of sleep disruptions, the black belt, the boss level if you will. It's not just about having difficulty falling asleep; it's about struggling to stay asleep, waking up too early, and then facing the day with impaired functioning. According to the Sleep Council, 25% of perimenopausal women in the UK meet the clinical criteria for insomnia. That's one in four women who are not just losing sleep but are

experiencing a level of sleep deprivation that could seriously affect their quality of life.

This affects millions of women and making insomnia not just a personal issue but a public health concern.

If you're part of this 25%, you're part of a significant subset of women who are likely struggling with the same sleepless nights and groggy mornings.

Insomnia isn't a once-in-a-while issue; it's a chronic problem that can persist for months or even years. Imagine running a marathon every day without adequate rest; that's what chronic insomnia can feel like. It's a long-term issue that requires long-term solutions.

The impact of insomnia goes beyond mere tiredness. It can affect your cognitive abilities, your emotional well-being, and even your physical health. Studies have linked chronic insomnia to a range of health issues, from depression and anxiety to an increased risk of heart disease and diabetes.

Self-Help Strategies

Cognitive Behavioural Therapy for Insomnia (CBT-I): This evidence-based approach helps you identify and change thought patterns and behaviours that contribute to insomnia. It's considered the first-line treatment for chronic insomnia.

Pharmacological Options: While medication should generally be a last resort, there are pharmaceutical options available for treating insomnia, such as sleep aids. However, these are usually recommended for short-term use only, due to the potential for dependency.

Consult a Healthcare Provider: If insomnia is affecting your quality of life, it's crucial to consult a healthcare provider for a thorough evaluation, which may include sleep studies and other diagnostic tests, and to discuss treatment options tailored to your needs.

Insomnia is a complex issue with multiple layers, but understanding its prevalence, impact, and potential solutions can empower you to take the steps needed to improve your sleep and, by extension, your overall well-being.

If you have *'The UncompliKated Perimenopause Journal'* there is a space to track your sleep every day. This is really important as you can start to see a potential correlation between the amount of sleep you get and your perimenopause symptoms.

The Energy Drain

The Energy Drain is that pesky culprit that sneaks in and steals your get-up-and-go. Yes, you've read that right; it's not your imagination or the Monday blues that last all week. A survey by Nuffield Health reveals that 72% of perimenopausal women in the UK are sailing on the same sluggish boat. This fatigue isn't a sign that you're morphing into a sloth; it's often a by-product of poor sleep quality. So, how can we pump some vitality back into your life without resorting to intravenous coffee?

Firstly, let's clarify something: we're talking about quality over quantity here. You could sleep for a solid eight hours and still wake up feeling like you've been through a spin cycle. That's because your sleep may not be hitting the deeper, restorative stages it needs to actually refresh you. Therefore, the focus should be on improving sleep quality.

Self-Help Strategies

Sleep Hygiene: Go all-in on influencing a beautiful night's sleep. Remember, you can't control how much sleep you get, but you can influence the number of hours you are in bed, and the quality of the sleep you might expect. Turn off all devices at least an hour before bed, create a beautiful self-care routine, and ensure that your room is the right temperature and is softly-lit before getting into bed.

Regular Exercise: You might think, "Exercise? I barely have the energy to lift the remote!" But hear me out. According to a study published in *PLOS ONE*, moderate aerobic exercise can significantly improve sleep quality. The trick is not to do it too close to bedtime, or you'll wind up revving your engines when you should be cooling your jets. **Approximately 2** hours before bed time should be the finishing point for exercise. Aim for at least thirty minutes a day of moderate exercise like walking, swimming, or yoga. Not only will it boost your mood, but it could also give you that much-needed energy kick.

Good Nutrition: Energy-boosting foods like bananas, quinoa, and lean proteins can be your best friends during this time. A well-balanced diet rich in vitamins and minerals supports not just your energy levels but your overall health. For instance, B vitamins are key for energy metabolism. Tuck into foods rich in B12, like fish and eggs, to help keep fatigue at bay.

Hydration: Dehydration is a notorious energy zapper. In a study from the *Journal of Nutrition,* even mild dehydration led to significant reductions in mood and cognitive performance. So, don't forget to hydrate throughout the day. And by hydrate, I don't mean topping up your coffee cup; plain water is your best bet.

Break the Caffeine Cycle: It's tempting to fight fire with fire by downing cups of coffee, but excessive caffeine can disrupt sleep and lead to an even bigger energy slump later on. A study in the *Journal of Clinical Sleep Medicine* found that consuming caffeine even six hours before bed can significantly disrupt sleep.

Mindfulness and Relaxation Techniques: Mindfulness meditation and deep-breathing exercises can improve sleep quality, according to the *Journal of Sleep Research*. Set aside a few minutes each day for deep breathing or a quick mindfulness session. This can help your body and mind relax, thereby improving the quality of your sleep.

Consult a Healthcare Provider: If all else fails and you're still dragging yourself through the day, it's time to consult a healthcare provider. Persistent fatigue could be a sign of other issues like anaemia or thyroid problems. Blood tests can rule these out and help guide further treatment.

Remember, a little humour and a lot of self-care can go a long way in managing perimenopausal symptoms like fatigue. This stage of life may be a bumpy ride, but with the right strategies, you can buckle up and make it less of a drag. And let's be real, once you've conquered the energy drain, what can't you do? So, hang in there, because you're stronger than you think, and there's a whole army of women (and healthcare providers) who've got your back.

The Perimenopausal Motivation Mystery: Where Did My Drive Go?

Motivation is that elusive spark that propels us to achieve our goals, tackle our to-do lists, and seize the day. But what happens when that spark fizzles out, leaving you feeling more like a damp squib than a firework? Welcome to the perimenopausal motivation mystery, where your get-up-and-go has got-up-and-gone. In this part of the chapter, we'll explore the reasons behind this lack of motivation and offer some practical solutions to reignite your inner drive. So, let's dive in, shall we?

If you find yourself lacking the motivation to do even the simplest tasks, you're not alone. According to a study by the British Menopause Society, up to 40% of perimenopausal women report a decrease in motivation. In the US, the numbers are slightly higher, with 45% of perimenopausal women experiencing a motivation slump.

Again, when we talk about such a large percentage (40-45%) of perimenopausal women in the UK experiencing a lack of motivation, we're talking about millions of women. That's a significant portion of the

THE UNCOMPLIKATED GUIDE TO PERIMENOPAUSE

population who are struggling to find the drive to accomplish their daily tasks, let alone chase their dreams.

If you're experiencing this motivation drain, you're part of a large group of women who are likely feeling the same way. It's like being a member of a club where the entry requirement is feeling 'meh' about life.

Many women report that this lack of motivation is a persistent issue, affecting them on a daily or even hourly basis. It's not just a fleeting feeling; it's a chronic state of being.

The repercussions of a lack of motivation are far-reaching. It can affect your career, your relationships, and even your mental health. A chronic lack of motivation can lead to feelings of inadequacy, depression, and a decreased quality of life.

The Causes
Hormonal Fluctuations: The hormonal changes during perimenopause can affect neurotransmitters like dopamine, which plays a key role in motivation.

Sleep Deprivation: As we discussed in the previous chapter, sleep disruptions are common during perimenopause, and lack of sleep can significantly impact your motivation levels.

Stress and Anxiety: The perimenopausal phase often comes with increased stress and anxiety, which can drain your emotional reserves and leave you feeling unmotivated.

Self-Help Strategies

Set Small Goals: Sometimes, the thought of a big task can be overwhelming. Breaking it down into smaller, more manageable tasks can make it easier to get started.

Seek Support: Whether it's talking to a friend, family member, or healthcare provider, some-times discussing your feelings can provide the emotional boost you need.

Consult a Healthcare Provider: If a lack of motivation is severely impacting your quality of life, it may be time to seek professional help. This could include counselling, medication, or hormone replacement therapy (HRT).

Lack of motivation during perimenopause can feel like you're stuck in a never-ending loop of "I can't be bothered." But remember, you're not alone, and this too shall pass. With the right strategies and a bit of support, you can find your lost motivation and get back to being the go-getter you know you are. So, while perimenopause may have stolen your mojo, it doesn't mean you can't steal it back.

Navigating Fatigue during Perimenopause

Time for a deep dive into the nuanced experience of fatigue that often punctuates the perimenopausal journey, providing you with a compass to navigate these changing tides with grace, wisdom, and resilience. As Chinese philosopher Lao Tzu once said,

"A journey of a thousand miles begins with a single step."

Let us take that step together, equipping ourselves with knowledge, empathy, and a spirit of solidarity as we venture through the multi-faceted landscape of perimenopause.

Fatigue during perimenopause is a complex tapestry woven from various threads that embody hormonal fluctuations, physical changes, and emotional shifts. Here, we unravel each thread, offering you a comprehensive understanding and actionable insights to not only manage fatigue but to flourish and thrive during this transformative period.

The Causes

Hormonal Fluctuations: At the heart of perimenopause lie the inevitable hormonal fluctuations, chiefly involving oestrogen and progesterone. These hormonal oscillations can significantly influence your sleep patterns, mood, and energy levels, creating a ripple effect that permeates various aspects of your well-being. It is essential to be aware of these changes, adopting a proactive approach to maintain a harmonious hormonal balance. Strategies such as consulting with healthcare providers for hormone therapy or integrating natural supplements can sometimes offer a beacon of relief during turbulent times.

Sleep Disturbances: During perimenopause, the sanctity of sleep can sometimes be elusive. Sleep disturbances, ranging from difficulty in falling asleep to frequent nocturnal awakenings, can exacerbate fatigue. The National Sleep Foundation suggests cultivating a serene sleeping environment, accompanied by a consistent bedtime routine, can pave the path to restorative sleep. Meditation and relaxation techniques can also serve as invaluable allies in your quest for restful slumber.

Hot Flashes and Night Sweats: Hot flashes and night sweats, the unwelcome companions of many women during perimenopause, can significantly disrupt your sleep, leading to a cascade of daytime fatigue. It might be helpful to dress in thermoregulating bamboo layers and keep your bedroom cool to mitigate these symptoms. Moreover, maintaining a well-hydrated state can sometimes dampen the intensity of hot flashes, allowing you to reclaim your comfort and tranquillity during the night.

I have created some CBT exercises to help with hot flashes and night sweats in *The UncompliKated Perimenopause Workbook'* that are a good starting point as. For some of you, HRT isn't an option or your preferred option, but regardless of whether you are going down the HRT route, CBT exercises can help make them much less severed.

Mood Disorders: Perimenopause can sometimes be a breeding ground for mood disorders, including bouts of depression or anxiety. These emotional upheavals can further contribute to disrupted sleep and heightened fatigue. Over 20% of women experience mood swings during perimenopause. It becomes imperative to foster emotional well-being through practices such as mindfulness, coaching, and fostering a supportive social network.

Metabolic Changes: As you journey through perimenopause, you might notice a slowdown in your metabolic rate, which can potentially contribute to weight gain and an increased sense of sluggishness. I recommend embracing a balanced diet rich in fibre, proteins, and healthy fats to support your metabolic health. Incorporating regular physical activity can also ignite your metabolic fires, infusing your days with enhanced vitality.

Chronic Stress: The perimenopausal phase might coincide with a surge in chronic stress, attributed to various life events like caregiving for aging parents or witnessing children leaving the nest. This added stress burden can significantly contribute to fatigue. Consider adopting stress management strategies such as yoga, meditation, and breathing exercises to foster a serene and balanced mind.

Nutritional Deficiencies: Nutritional deficiencies can often lurk in the background, silently contributing to dwindling energy levels. It becomes vital to ensure a nutritionally rich diet that fortifies your body with essential vitamins and minerals. Regular health check-ups can help in identifying and addressing any nutritional gaps, allowing you to maintain a robust energy reservoir.

Decreased Physical Activity: During this transitional phase, you might find it somewhat challenging to maintain the same vigour in your physical activities, which in turn, can lead to dwindling energy levels. Yet, as Edward Stanley noted, "Those who think they have not time for bodily exercise will sooner or later have to find time for illness." There-fore, it's crucial to rekindle your kinetic spirit, maybe through gentle exercises like yoga or Pilates, which not only revitalise your body but also rejuvenate your mind. Even a daily walk, bathed in the gentle em-brace of nature, can serve as a potent antidote to fatigue.

Pain and Physical Discomfort: Perimenopausal women sometimes en-counter an increase in physical discomfort and pain, stemming from hormonal fluctuations. This not only hampers daily activities but can also usher in a pervasive sense of fatigue. Finding relief might involve exploring various therapeutic avenues, from acupuncture to massage therapy, which can potentially alleviate physical distress, fostering a sense of bodily harmony and well-being.

Changes in Thyroid Function: Thyroid function can sometimes veer off its regular course during perimenopause, contributing significantly to fatigue. Periodic screenings can help in monitoring thyroid health, fa-cilitating timely interventions if necessary. Nutrition also plays a pivotal role, with a diet rich in iodine, selenium, and zinc being instrumental in supporting thyroid function.

Altered Blood Sugar Levels: Hormonal changes can sometimes wreak havoc on insulin sensitivity and blood sugar levels, resulting in fluctua-tions in energy throughout the day. Embracing a diet with low glycae-mic index foods can help in maintaining glycaemic harmony, ensuring a steady energy supply and keeping fatigue at bay.

Decreased Resilience to Illness: During perimenopause, your immune resilience might somewhat diminish, making it slightly harder to bounce back from illnesses. This can further add layers to existing fatigue. It thus becomes essential to bolster your immune fortress through a nu-tritious diet, adequate sleep, and stress management, fostering an en-vironment of vitality and robust health.

Cognitive Changes: Cognitive shifts are another facet of perimenopause, with some women experiencing memory lapses or difficulty concentrating. These changes can be mentally draining, contributing to a sense of fatigue. Engaging in cognitive exercises, mindfulness practices, and ensuring adequate omega-3 fatty acids in your diet can sometimes aid in enhancing cognitive function, steering you through this changing landscape with grace and agility. See more in chapter 9.

Alterations in Red Blood Cell Production: Hormonal fluctuations might influence the production of red blood cells, potentially affecting energy levels. Ensuring an iron-rich diet can sometimes help in optimising red blood cell production, serving as a vital source of energy and vitality.

Vitamin D Deficiency: Vitamin D deficiency is a common concern during perimenopause, often contributing to fatigue and low energy levels. Regular sunlight exposure and including vitamin D-rich foods in your diet can potentially uplift your energy levels, acting as rays of sunshine in your perimenopausal journey.

Self-Help Strategies

Incorporate Vitamin B-Rich Foods: Opt for whole grains, leafy greens, and fish to give your body the Vitamin B it craves for better energy management.

Fuel Up on Iron: Lentils, spinach, and poultry can be excellent sources of iron, vital for fighting off fatigue.

Regular Exercise: Yes, it sounds counterproductive when you're already tired, but even a brisk twenty-minute walk can do wonders for your energy levels.

Choose the Right Time to Exercise: Opt for a time when you usually feel a bit more energetic, so it doesn't feel like a chore.

Stay Hydrated: Often fatigue is just thirst in disguise. Make sure you're drinking enough water throughout the day.

Mindfulness and Breathing Techniques: A mere five to ten minutes of focused breathing or mindfulness meditation can be a real game-changer for your emotional well-being.

Stress Management: Identify stress triggers and find healthy coping mechanisms, be it a hobby, talking to friends, or professional counselling.

Get Quality Sleep: Make your bedroom a sleep sanctuary. Dim the lights, keep it cool, and banish electronic devices at least an hour before bedtime.

Consider Short Naps: A fifteen-to-twenty-minute power nap can recharge your batteries without leaving you groggy.

Consult a Healthcare Provider: If your fatigue persists or worsens, seek medical advice. You may need tests to rule out other underlying conditions like anaemia or thyroid issues.

Track Your Symptoms: Use a journal or an app to note when your fatigue is at its worst. This data can be very helpful for your healthcare provider.

Connect with Support Groups: Sometimes sharing experiences and tips with others going through the same thing can be incredibly empowering. My Facebook group 'Perimenopause with Kate Grosvenor' is there for you if you wish to join.

Limit Caffeine and Alcohol: These can mess with your sleep quality, thus perpetuating the fatigue cycle.

Take Breaks: When doing tasks or at work, short and frequent breaks can help in maintaining energy levels throughout the day. The Pomodoro Technique is great for encouraging you to do this.

By implementing these strategies, you're not just putting up a fight against fatigue; you're sculpting a lifestyle that champions vitality. You've got this!

> *"She was powerful, not because she wasn't scared,*
> *but because she went on strongly, despite the fear."*
> **Atticus Poetry**

Let this be our guiding philosophy as we navigate the complex yet enriching journey of perimenopause, turning each challenge into an opportunity for growth, transformation, and rejuvenation.

But, most of all, my darling girl, rest when you need to rest.

Sleep if you're overly tired.

Let's not act like superwomen with a never-ending supply of energy. This is a time to be compassionate, considerate and kind to ourselves. I highly recommend a twenty-to-thirty-minute nap in the afternoon to refresh and restore our energy supplies. I promise you, from the bottom of my heart, that it won't cause the world to stop spinning. Everyone will manage without you while you rest.

CHAPTER 20

Feeling Creaky?

The lowdown on your changing muscles and joints

If you've ever woken up feeling like you've just completed an Ironman triathlon – minus the training, the cheering crowds, and the sense of accomplishment – you might be experiencing the musculoskeletal changes that often accompany perimenopause. From joint pain to muscle aches, these symptoms can make you feel like you're aging in dog years. But don't despair; you're not alone, and there are ways to manage these changes. So, let's roll up our sleeves (carefully, to avoid any shoulder issues) and dive in.

Joint Pain

Joint pain during perimenopause can be likened to that: omnipresent, inconvenient and – let's be honest – annoying. According to the NHS, up to 60% of perimenopausal women experience joint pain. That's a lot of women who may be putting their hands on their hips not just to make a point, but also because it hurts less than leaving them hanging by their sides.

The Causes

As with many symptoms during this life stage, the decrease in oestrogen plays a major role in joint pain. Oestrogen acts as a natural lubricant for your joints. So, when levels decline, it's like running your car with less oil; things get creaky.

Oestrogen Decline: The primary cause, leading to reduced lubrication and more friction in the joints.

Inflammation: Lower levels of oestrogen can cause inflammation, contributing to pain.

Weight Gain: The added pounds can put more stress on your joints, particularly the knees and hips.

Lifestyle Factors: Lack of exercise and poor diet can worsen the condition.

Self-Help Strategies

Regular Exercise: Low-impact exercises like swimming, cycling, or walking can keep those joints moving without adding more stress. According to the Arthritis Foundation, just 150 minutes of moderate exercise per week can improve your mobility and decrease pain. Even if you're groaning at the very thought of moving that achy knee, remember – motion is lotion!

Anti-Inflammatory Diet: Dietary changes can be powerful. Omega-3 fatty acids, found in fish like salmon and in flaxseeds, can help combat inflammation. Various studies suggest that a diet rich in omega-3 fatty acids can reduce joint pain severity in the morning and improve joint functionality. You can't go wrong with a salmon dinner, can you?

Turmeric: This golden spice is known for its anti-inflammatory properties. Some studies indicate that it can be as effective as some anti-inflammatory drugs.

Ginger: A staple in natural medicine, ginger has been shown to have anti-inflammatory effects similar to ibuprofen and COX-2 inhibitors.

Glucosamine and Chondroitin: These are naturally occurring compounds that may help with joint pain, though scientific opinions are mixed.

**Always consult a healthcare provider before taking any supplements, especially if you are already on medication.

Consult a Healthcare Provider: If your joint pain is more persistent than a bad soap opera storyline, it's probably time to get professional help. Various treatments, from physiotherapy to medication, can provide relief.

Joint pain might be an unwelcome guest during perimenopause, but that doesn't mean you can't show it the door – or at least get it to behave. Being proactive with exercise, diet, and, if necessary, medical intervention can help you navigate this period with less groaning and more grace.

Muscle Tension

If you've ever thought you'd look great draped in heavy jewellery, be careful what you wish for. Muscle tension can feel like you're wearing the world's heaviest necklace, except it's made of stress, hormones, and perhaps a sprinkle of 'life,' for good measure. While there are no official UK statistics on perimenopausal muscle tension, many women during this phase would likely volunteer themselves as case studies.

The Causes

In terms of what's pulling your strings – or rather, your muscles – several culprits are at play:

Hormonal Fluctuations: Hormones don't only have a VIP pass to your emotions; they also affect your muscles. As hormone levels fluctuate, this can lead to increased muscle tension.

Stress:. Stress exacerbates muscle tension, making your muscles a battleground for hormonal and emotional warfare.

Physical Inactivity: It's a bit of a catch-22; you're tense, so you move less, but moving less makes you even more tense.

Poor Posture: Hours of slouching at a desk or over a smartphone can further stress muscles, making them more susceptible to tension.

Self-Help Strategies
Stretching: Regular stretching is like giving your muscles a good old pat on the back, saying, "There, there, it'll be all right." Not just any random stretches will do, though. Focus on targeted stretching exercises that work on your neck, back, and shoulders. According to the American College of Sports Medicine, stretching at least two times a week can significantly improve muscle tension.

Heat Therapy: If you've ever felt the urge to become a mermaid and live the rest of your life in warm water, this one's for you. Warm baths, hot water bottles, or heat packs can offer temporary relief from muscle tension. Studies have shown that heat therapy can improve blood flow and relax muscles, offering a twofold benefit.

Lavender Oil: Known for its relaxation properties, some people find that massaging diluted lavender oil onto tense areas can offer relief.

Magnesium Supplements: Often referred to as the 'relaxation mineral,' magnesium can help muscles relax. However, it's essential to consult your healthcare provider before diving into the supplement aisle, especially as there are several different types of magnesium.

Chamomile Tea: While it's not as direct as applying heat or stretching, sipping on chamomile tea is thought to have muscle-relaxant properties.

Consult a Healthcare Provider: For those stubborn muscles that refuse to loosen up, even after you've tried all the DIY tricks, it might be time for some professional intervention. A healthcare provider may recommend muscle relaxants or refer you to a physical therapist who specialises in muscle tension treatment. They may even offer diagnostic tests to rule out other underlying issues.

Carrying the world on your shoulders might make you a superhero in the eyes of those around you, but even superheroes need a break. Implementing self-care techniques like stretching, heat therapy, and possibly natural remedies could turn that heavy necklace of tension into a more manageable accessory. And if all else fails, professional help is just a phone call away.

Frozen Shoulder

As children, the game of statues was a test of how well we could stand frozen in time. Fast-forward a few decades, and some of us are stuck playing an involuntary, grown-up version, also known as 'frozen shoulder.' With the *British Journal of General Practice* highlighting that the incidence of this condition peaks between the ages of 40 and 60, it's no wonder perimenopausal women are joining the ranks of involuntary statue impersonators.

The Causes

Doctor Knows Best, Except When They Don't: The exact causes of frozen shoulder are as elusive as a teenager avoiding chores. However, certain factors contributing to it have been identified:

Hormonal Changes: Ah, hormones again. They're the uninvited party guests that spill drinks everywhere – in this case, affecting joint mobility.

Reduced Physical Activity: A sedentary lifestyle is about as good for your shoulders as a snowstorm is for a beach party.

Stress: Stress doesn't only tighten your facial muscles into a well-practised scowl; it might also be restricting your shoulder movements.

Other Medical Conditions: Conditions like diabetes and cardiovascular diseases have also been linked to frozen shoulder, turning it into a sort of medical edition Cluedo 'who-done-it.'

Self-Help Strategies

Physical Therapy: Stiff shoulders need encouragement, much like a shy person at a dance. Physical therapy, consisting of exercises to improve your range of motion, can be a game-changer. According to the American Physical Therapy Association, more than 50% of patients saw improvement with targeted exercises.

Pain Management: Pain management is essential when you're wincing every time you reach for the top shelf. Over-the-counter pain relievers like ibuprofen can offer temporary relief, allowing you to get the most out of physical therapy. However, it's crucial to consult your healthcare provider before starting any new medication.

Heat Packs: Like a warm hug to your shoulder, heat packs can offer temporary relief by improving blood flow to the affected area.

Turmeric: Curcumin, the active component in turmeric, is known for its anti-inflammatory properties. Some people find mixing a teaspoonful in warm milk helps, but this isn't proven in the context of frozen shoulder.

Consult a Healthcare Provider: When all else fails, a healthcare provider may offer advanced solutions like corticosteroid injections for severe inflammation. For extreme cases that don't respond to other treatments, surgery might even be recommended to break up the joint capsule. In other words, the big guns.

While a frozen shoulder won't win you any games of statues, it's crucial to take action to regain your range of motion. Physical therapy can act as the choreographer teaching your shoulder new dance moves, while pain management and perhaps natural remedies might offer relief from the discomfort. And never underestimate the expertise of a healthcare provider; they could just be the one to thaw your frozen shoulder.

So, don't stay frozen in discomfort. Take proactive steps to ease the symptoms, and with some persistence, your shoulder could be ready to break free from its statue routine.

Muscle Aches

There's tired, and then there's, "Your muscles are so sore you'd swear you were the main course in an elephant stampede" tired. Take solace in knowing you're far from alone in this sore ensemble.

The Causes

Hormones, Again? Yes, your hormones are again doing that thing where they forget they're supposed to make you feel good. Fluctuations in hormone levels can mess with muscle function like a poorly tuned piano – sounding off and causing discomfort.

Sluggish Lifestyle: If your exercise routine has been reduced to lifting the remote, your muscles might protest when asked to do anything more strenuous.

You Are What You Eat: Poor nutrition can make your muscles groan louder than a an old wooden floorboard in a haunted house. A lack of essential nutrients can lead to muscle fatigue and soreness.

Self-Help Strategies

Regular Exercise: Let's not go running a marathon just yet, but a bit of aerobic exercise, combined with strength training, can kick those muscle aches to the curb. According to the National Institute for Health

and Care Excellence (NICE), moderate exercise has been shown to reduce the risk of chronic muscle pain by up to 25%.

Nutrition: Feeding your muscles is as important as watering a plant.
Adequate protein intake can keep your muscles robust, while foods rich
in magnesium and potassium can help with muscle function. According
to the NHS, women aged 19 to 64 need about 45g of protein a day. So,
consider adding lean meats, fish, eggs, or plant-based options like tofu
to your menu.

Epsom Salt Baths: The magnesium in Epsom salts is absorbed through
the skin, helping to relax muscles.

Cherry Juice: Some studies indicate that the antioxidants in cherry juice
can reduce muscle inflammation.

Consult a Healthcare Provider: If your muscles are still sending you
'SOS' signals, consult a healthcare provider. They might recommend
treatments ranging from medication to massage therapy, effectively
making you less of a human stress ball.

Muscle aches during perimenopause might make you feel like an old,
creaky door hinge, but the good news is you're not due for a breakdown.
Just as you would oil that hinge, your body needs its maintenance too.

So, the next time you feel like you've been trampled by a herd of metaphorical elephants, remember that you have the tools to shake off the
dust and rise. As the saying goes, "A smooth sea never made a skilled
sailor." Similarly, navigating through the aches and pains of perimenopause can make you the captain of your own well-being.

CHAPTER 21

Hot Flushes & Cold Truths

The vasomotor variety show

L et's chat about something that might be turning up the heat (or sometimes cooling it down unexpectedly) in your day-to-day lives. We're talking about vasomotor symptoms: the sudden climatic shifts occurring within our splendid bodies.

Hot Flushes/Flashes

Imagine you've just become the proud owner of an internal tropical climate – a touch of the Maldives, right in the comfort of your own body. Hot flushes, the well-renowned heat waves that embrace you out of nowhere, are practically a rite of passage, gracing around 75% of women in the perimenopause transition.

In essence, hot flushes are the rave parties that your hormones throw, and it seems they do love a good bash quite frequently during perimenopause. The primary cause behind these events is the fluctuating levels of oestrogen in your body. As the oestrogen level takes a bit of a roller coaster ride, it tends to affect the hypothalamus, the part of the brain responsible for regulating body temperature.

When the hypothalamus gets a bit muddled due to these hormonal fluctuations, it sometimes thinks the body is too hot and triggers a hot flash to cool things down. This causes your heart rate to increase, blood vessels to dilate (hello, rosy cheeks!), and sweat glands to go into overdrive to cool you down, even when there wasn't actually a need to.

Apart from hormonal fluctuations, here are a few other factors that might cause or exacerbate hot flashes during perimenopause:

The Causes

Stress: High-stress levels can sometimes be a VIP guest at these hot flash parties. Try to keep stress at bay to avoid triggering these heat surges.

Diet and Lifestyle: Consuming spicy foods, alcohol or caffeine can sometimes set the stage for a hot flash performance.

Smoking: Yes, it's not just bad for your lungs; smoking can invite more frequent and severe hot flashes due to its effect on oestrogen levels.

Obesity: Carrying excess weight can increase the likelihood of experiencing hot flashes. Keeping a healthy weight might tone down the frequency and intensity of these episodes.

Genetic Factors: If your mum or your sister were the life of the hot flash party, you might be predisposed to be the star of such parties too.

Medications: Certain medications can have side effects that include hot flashes. If you suspect your medication is playing the DJ at these heat parties, you might want to have a chat with your doctor about it.

Environmental Factors: Sometimes, a warm room or a change in the weather can trigger a hot flash. You might find yourself being more sensitive to environmental temperatures during perimenopause.

Hot flashes might make you feel like you're auditioning for a one-woman show called 'The Human Furnace,' but fear not, there are ways to manage these steamy episodes.

Self-Help Strategies

Dress in Layers: As any savvy dresser will tell you, layers are not just a fashion statement – they're a hot flash strategy. Lightweight, breathable fabrics can be your best friends. When a hot flash strikes, you can peel off a layer faster than you'd say, "Is it hot in here, or is it just me?"

Hydrate: Staying hydrated might sound like a cure-all for everything, but it really does help manage hot flashes. Cold water can act as your internal air conditioner.

Mindfulness and Breathing Exercises: According to the National Institute of Health and Care Excellence (NICE), cognitive behavioural therapy (CBT) techniques, like mindfulness and deep-breathing exercises, can reduce hot flash severity for some women by up to 40%.

Phytoestrogens: Foods rich in phytoestrogens such as soybeans, tofu, and flaxseeds have been shown to reduce the frequency of hot flashes in some studies. However, the research is inconclusive and could vary from person to person.

Black Cohosh: This herb is often cited for its potential to relieve hot flashes, although medical opinion is divided on its efficacy. If you're considering black cohosh, it's best to consult your healthcare provider first.

Evening Primrose Oil: While not universally supported by scientific evidence, some women find relief by using evening primrose oil.

Sage: Some women swear by sage tea for hot flash relief. It's worth a try, and at the very least, you'll have a delicious, calming cuppa.

Vitamin E: Supplementing with Vitamin E has shown some promise in reducing the severity of hot flashes, although it's always a good idea to check with a healthcare provider before starting any new supplement regimen.

See the chapter at the back of this book for more information on supplements.

Hot flashes might make you feel like you're living in a perpetual heatwave, but there are plenty of strategies and natural remedies to help you keep your cool. After all, this phase of life isn't just about survival; it's about thriving. So, whether you're peeling off layers or sipping on sage tea, remember, you've got this.

Night Sweats

When you wake up feeling like you've run a marathon in a tropical rainforest, you know it's not just a case of 'sleeping hot.' Night sweats can be one of the most disruptive symptoms of perimenopause. But don't sweat it (pun absolutely intended); there are ways to get a good night's rest.

Self-Help Strategies

Breathable Bedding: Swap out those heavy duvets for lightweight, moisture-wicking sheets and blankets. Consider fabrics like bamboo, cotton, or specialised wicking materials that pull moisture away from your skin. Bamboo is my personal favourite because it just doesn't seem to get damp and 'heavy' the way that even cotton does.

Sleepwear Choices: Investing in moisture-wicking sleepwear can also make a difference. Pyjamas made from breathable materials will help you sleep comfortably and reduce those night sweats. Bamboo for the win again here!

Keep It Cool: A fan on your nightstand or a portable air conditioner can work wonders. You might not be able to control your internal thermostat, but you can certainly adjust the room's temperature.

Side Note: I have one next to my bed, on my dressing table, so I have a fighting chance of getting my make-up to set, and a quiet one on my desk in case I'm hot flushing when I'm on a zoom call.

Hydration: Keep a glass of cold water by your bedside. When a night sweat strikes, hydrating can help you cool down quickly. Some women even swear by a hot water bottle filled with ice water!

Monitor Eating and Drinking Habits: Spicy foods and alcohol can trigger hot flashes and night sweats. If you notice a pattern, try altering your evening meals to see if that makes a difference.

Carry a Spritz Bottle: Whether it's an aerosol can of Evian spritz, or a refillable bottle, just having a little refresh during the day (or night) can work wonders for just feeling more comfortable.

Cooling Pillows: The jury is a little bit out on the effectiveness of these but hey, if you're really struggling at night time, I would genuinely throw everything you have at this to allow for better sleep.

Herbal Teas: Certain herbal teas like chamomile and valerian root are known for their calming effects and might help you sleep through the night sweat-free. However, always consult your healthcare provider when introducing new herbs into your regimen.

Magnesium Supplements: There are studies suggest that magnesium supplements can help with night sweats. Always consult a healthcare provider before adding new supplements to your routine, though.

Flaxseeds: Rich in phytoestrogens, flaxseeds may offer some relief from night sweats. Try adding them to your evening smoothie or yoghurt.

Trying adding them to overnight oats too with Greek yoghurt for an amazing morning boost.

Acupuncture: Though scientific support is mixed; some women report that acupuncture helps in reducing night sweats. If you're open to alternative therapies, it might be worth a shot.

Remember, while night sweats can be uncomfortable and disruptive, they're not insurmountable. With some proactive steps and perhaps a few natural remedies, you can improve your chances of a good night's sleep. After all, Shakespeare said,

"Sleep . . . knits up the ravelled sleave of care."

Let's ensure your 'sleave of care' is as comfortable as possible, shall we?

Cold Flashes

You're all geared up for hot flashes and you've prepared like a pro. Your cooling pillows are in place, your fan's oscillating like a well-oiled machine, and you've got your spritz bottle at the ready. But then, out of nowhere, you're hit with the chills. It's like expecting a fastball and getting a knuckleball instead. The universe has a cheeky sense of humour, doesn't it?

While hot flashes get all the media attention, cold flashes are like the introverted cousin who only speaks when spoken to. Cold flashes are less understood, but they often occur as a quick, unexpected drop in body temperature. Sometimes this can be a counter-reaction to a hot flash, or it may happen independently. Hormonal fluctuations during perimenopause get the blame again, causing your internal thermostat to go a bit haywire.

Self-Help Strategies

Layer Up, Layer Down: One minute you're hot, and the next you're not. Dress in layers so you can easily add or remove clothing as your body's temperature dictates.

Drink Warm Liquids: Have a flask of herbal tea or hot water nearby. When a cold flash strikes, a warm drink can provide quick comfort. Go for caffeine-free options to avoid triggering any hot flashes in retaliation.

Room Temperature: Since your own internal thermostat is acting up, focus on controlling the room's climate. A small space heater can quickly warm a room and is easy to turn off when the heat is back on. I use the little oil-filled radiators in the attic bedrooms as they are more budget-friendly.

Mindful Breathing: Believe it or not, focused, deep breathing can help regulate your body temperature. Try taking slow, deep breaths in through the nose and out through the mouth when you feel a cold flash coming on.

Ginger Tea: Ginger is known for its warming properties. A nice cup of ginger tea can be a great way to combat a cold flash.

Warm Compress: A warm compress or heating pad can offer immediate relief. Keep one handy in your living room or office for quick access.

Stay Active: Physical activity gets the blood flowing, which naturally raises body temperature. If you can, a few minutes of light exercise could ward off the chill.

Sadly, cold flashes aren't as well-studied as hot flashes, which makes it difficult to present a statistical breakdown of their frequency. However, anecdotal reports suggest that a significant number of women experience them to some degree.

Cold flashes may not have the notoriety of hot flashes, but they offer their own unique form of discomfort. Thankfully, they're also manageable. So, whether you're breaking into a spontaneous sweat or clutching a hot water bottle for dear life, remember this too shall pass. After all, variety is the spice of life – even if it comes in temperature swings!

As we gently close this chapter, let's take a moment to appreciate our magnificent bodies for their adaptability and resilience. These vasomotor symptoms are just transient guests, visiting us during this vibrant journey of transformation.

CHAPTER 22

Ear We Go Again!

Finding your balance in the wobbly world of perimenopause

If you've ever felt like you're starring in your own version of a slapstick comedy – tripping over invisible obstacles, bumping into walls, or feeling like you're on a merry-go-round when you're standing still – you're not alone. Welcome to the world of perimenopausal ears, balance, and spatial awareness. It's a world that can be disorienting, to say the least, but it's also one that's surprisingly common. So, let's delve into this labyrinth of symptoms and explore ways to find your footing again.

Dizzy Spells

So, you're going about your day, perhaps doing a bit of shopping, meeting up with friends, or tackling that bottomless laundry pile, when suddenly – whoa! You're not on a merry-go-round, but it sure feels like it. This is the dizzying world of perimenopausal vertigo. It's like the universe is trying to give you a surprise trip to Disneyland but forgot to ask if you like roller coasters.

As we're well aware, oestrogen is the star of the show – or rather the diva creating chaos during perimenopause. A decline in oestrogen levels can affect the inner ear, which is basically the body's spirit level. Now throw into the mix changes in blood sugar and blood pressure, and you've got a recipe for occasional dizziness. Around 30% of women according to NHS stats are joining this not-so-exclusive club.

Self-Help Strategies

Stay Hydrated: Remember, water is your best friend, even when you don't feel thirsty. Dehydration can make you feel like you're living in a perpetual tumble dryer cycle. Keep a refillable water bottle at your side at all times, and your inner ear might just thank you.

Eat Regularly: You'd be amazed what a packet of mixed nuts or a piece of fruit can do. Eating small meals throughout the day can help regulate blood sugar levels, which in turn can keep dizziness at bay. Try to aim for a balanced diet rich in protein, fibre, and good fats to keep your blood sugar steady.

Mind Your Posture: Sometimes a swift change in posture can send you into a spin. Make sure to get up slowly if you've been sitting or lying down for a long time. Trust me, your future non-dizzy self will thank you.

Herbal Remedies: Ginger is known for its anti-dizziness properties. A cup of ginger tea or even a ginger lozenge can help settle a spinning head.

Consult a Healthcare Provider: If you've tried the self-help strategies and still feel like you're auditioning for a tightrope act, it's time to get professional advice. Your doctor may recommend tests to rule out other under-lying conditions and could prescribe medication to help manage the symptoms.

Life in perimenopause is never dull, and dizzy spells just add another level of unpredictability to the mix. However, with a few lifestyle adjustments and maybe a bit of herbal assistance, you can keep your feet more firmly on the ground. After all, perimenopause may be a roller coaster, but who says you can't enjoy the ride – with both eyes open and a stable horizon in view?

Tinnitus

Let's talk about that uninvited guest that's been crashing your cranial party lately: Tinnitus. You know, the constant, high-pitched ringing or buzzing in your ears that seems to think it has an all-access pass to your personal soundscape. Well, you're not alone in wanting to show it the exit door. According to a UK study, about 10% of the population has to put up with tinnitus, and the numbers are even higher among perimenopausal women. It's like your ears are saying, "Oh, you think you've got enough on your plate? Here, have a side of relentless buzzing."

What's Ringing the Bell?

Just as with many other perimenopausal symptoms, our 'friend' oestrogen is once again playing tricks on us. Declining levels of this hormone can mess around with the inner ear, leading to that constant 'eeee' you might be hearing. As if that weren't enough, stress and high blood pressure are also known culprits. Yes, these too can add a layer of auditory 'fog' to your already packed hormonal landscape.

Self-Help Strategies

White Noise: You might not be able to stop the noise, but you can certainly drown it out. White noise machines or even white noise apps can fill your auditory field with something a bit more tolerable than the 'bzzzz' that's been dogging you.

Stress Management: While it might be tempting to stress about your stress, that could just turn the tinnitus volume knob higher. Mindfulness and deep breathing techniques can work wonders. A few deep breaths can bring your stress levels down, and might just take the edge off that ringing. If you're feeling adventurous, you might even try a gentle yoga class aimed at relaxation.

Herbal Remedies: Ginkgo biloba, a herbal supplement, has been suggested to improve blood circulation, potentially offering some relief from tinnitus. However, it's important to consult a healthcare provider before diving into herbal treatments, as they can interact with other medications you may be taking.

Consult an Audiologist: If your personal head concert won't stop, and you've tried all the DIY hacks with no luck, it might be time to consult an audiologist. They can provide targeted treatments and rule out other underlying conditions.

While tinnitus might feel like a noisy nuisance you'd rather not deal with, remember that there are ways to manage it. So next time your ears start playing their own drum, take a deep breath, turn on some soothing white noise, and remember: This too shall pass. Eventually, your ears should get the message and end the party, letting you get back to your life's soundtrack – buzz-free.

Vertigo

Vertigo is like that feeling when you step off a merry-go-round, and the world keeps spinning, only you don't want to. According to the NHS, roughly one in four women going through perimenopause experience vertigo. That's a fair number of us wobbling around like Weeble toy (do you remember those from the 70's? "Weebles wobble, but they don't fall down").

The Causes

Our hormonal merry-go-round (yes, it's hormones, yet again) has a direct impact on the vestibular system, which is in charge of your sense of balance and spatial orientation. When oestrogen levels dip and surge, it's like someone gave your inner gyroscope a good shake, leaving you feeling like you're navigating through a revolving door that just won't stop.

Self-Help Strategies

Vestibular Rehabilitation: Think of this as physical therapy for your balance. Vestibular rehabilitation involves specific exercises designed to improve your balance and reduce dizziness. Practising these exercises, often as simple as head movements or walking in a straight line, can help recalibrate your internal compass.

Avoid Triggers: You might be surprised at how certain elements in your diet can make a difference. Consumables like caffeine and alcohol might add a little extra spin to your already unstable world. Best to limit these if you're prone to bouts of vertigo.

Ginger Tea, Anyone? While not a cure-all, some natural remedies like ginger tea have been suggested to help with nausea that can accompany vertigo. In addition, hydration is key, as dehydration can make vertigo symptoms worse.

Consult a Healthcare Provider: If you're spinning more than a contestant on a game show, it's time to consult a healthcare provider. Accurate diagnosis and treatment options, including medications, can provide relief and may even offer a permanent exit off the dizzying ride of vertigo.

It's a bit disorienting when you feel like you're the centre of a spinning top. But, with the right strategies, you can stop the world and get off for a bit. And as you step off that merry-go-round, you'll find the world is a whole lot more manageable when it's not twirling around you.

Itchy Ears

When your ears are itchy, it's like they're trying to tell you something, but you just can't figure out what. It's not exactly the Morse code you were hoping to decode during perimenopause, is it? While there are no UK-wide statistics that can confirm how many of us are surreptitiously trying to scratch our ears while on a Zoom call, anecdotal evidence suggests that it's a pretty common irritation among perimenopausal women.

The Itchy and Scratchy Show – Inside Your Ears

What's behind this maddening itch? Once again, we can tip our hats to hormonal changes. Lower levels of oestrogen can lead to dry skin, and yes, that includes the inside of your ears. It's like they've become the Sahara Desert when you weren't looking.

Self-Help Strategies

Moisturise: Grab some natural oil like olive oil or coconut oil. A little dab on a cotton ball can go a long way in moisturising that delicate skin. Just be careful not to stick it too far into the ear canal – this isn't a treasure hunt.

Steer Clear of Cotton Swabs: You might be tempted to take a cotton swab and dig for gold but resist the urge. Cotton swabs can push earwax further into the ear canal, worsening the dryness and causing more itchiness – a viscous circle!

Natural Remedies: A drop or two of warm chamomile or tea tree oil has been known to bring relief due to their anti-inflammatory properties. Just make sure you're not allergic to these oils before you go pouring them into your ears.

Consult a Healthcare Provider: If you find that your ear itches are becoming as persistent as a door-to-door salesman, it's probably time to get some professional advice. In some cases, persistent itchiness can be a sign of an underlying condition that may need more targeted treatment.

Ear's to you (sorry, I couldn't help it!) my lovely, if you've been thinking your itchy ears are just a minor nuisance, you'll soon realise that even the little things can demand big attention. But don't worry, with a few simple strategies, you can make sure your ears stay as serene as a spa day. After all, they've got a lot of listening to do.

Nausea

Nausea is like morning sickness back for an encore. It's one of the weird symptoms I experienced which gave me a nudge to think that what was going on with me was hormonal (I had horrific morning sickness with all three of my girls). While I don't have specific UK stats to back this up, many women navigating the perimenopausal roller coaster report bouts of nausea.

The Causes

Hormonal Highs and Lows: The hormonal swings associated with perimenopause don't just affect your mood; they can wreak havoc on your gastrointestinal system too.

The Stress Connection: Let's not underestimate the power of stress, either. Stress can not only make you want to pull your hair out but can also kick your nausea up a notch. It's like a double-feature no one asked for.

Self-Help Strategies

Eat Small Meals: One of the best things you can do to keep nausea at bay is to eat small meals more frequently. It's a bit like giving your digestive system bite-sized snacks instead of a three-course meal. Little and often.

Dry Snacks: Things like water biscuits, rich tea biscuits, plain breadsticks, etc. seem to work really well to keep the nausea at bay too. Even try stem ginger biscuits, as you get the added help with the ginger.

Ginger Tea, Your New Best Friend: Ginger has been the go-to remedy for seasickness, morning sickness, and well, any kind of sickness, really, for ages. Brewing up some fresh ginger tea could be the tummy-taming trick you've been searching for.

Peppermint Oil: Inhaling peppermint oil can sometimes help with nausea. Just a couple of drops on a tissue held near your nose might do the trick. But be cautious, the scent can be potent – use it sparingly unless you want to smell like a walking Tic Tac.

Acupressure Wristbands: Widely available and relatively inexpensive, these wristbands apply pressure to specific points on your wrist that can help with nausea. They're like those friendship bracelets from back in the 80s, but with a purpose beyond aesthetics.

Consult a Healthcare Provider: If your nausea becomes the uninvited guest that overstays its welcome, consult a healthcare provider. This could be a symptom of something more serious or may require medication to manage effectively.

While nausea can be a pesky side effect of the hormonal merry-go-round that is perimenopause, it doesn't have to ruin the party. With a little preparation and the right remedies, you can keep those queasy feelings at bay and continue rocking on like the fabulous woman you are.

Sensitivity to Noise

Ever feel like the world has suddenly decided to host a rock concert in your living room without asking you? Sensitivity to noise is one of those symptoms that don't get the limelight, but it's surprisingly common during perimenopause.

The Causes

Hormonal Harmonics: You can thank your ever-fluctuating hormones for this newfound 'superpower.' Changes in hormonal levels can affect the way your brain processes auditory information, making you more sensitive to sound. It's like you've been given a new set of ears, but they're set to max volume.

Stress: The Silent Amplifier: Don't underestimate the role stress plays in amplifying your sensitivity to noise. When you're stressed, your senses are heightened, and you're more likely to find noise disturbing.

Stress may not have a volume knob, but it sure knows how to turn things up to 11.

Self-Help Strategies

Earplugs: The Barrier You Didn't Know You Needed: Earplugs might not be a fashion statement, but they're an effective way to reduce the noise levels around you. You can think of them as noise-cancelling headphones without the headphones.

Soundproof Your Sanctuary: If you find your home has become an cacophony of irksome noises, consider some soundproofing options. Heavy curtains, rugs, even strategically placed bookshelves can dampen sound. It's a bit like turning your home into a recording studio, only you're recording peace and quiet.

Mindfulness and Meditation: Mindfulness techniques can sometimes help you become less reactive to irritations like noise. Through mindfulness, you can learn to mentally 'step back' from the noise and observe it without letting it drive you up the wall.

White Noise Machines: A white noise machine can create a constant ambient sound, essentially helping to mask more jarring noises. It's a bit like fighting fire with fire, only quieter.

Consult a Healthcare Provider: If the cacophony becomes too unbearable, and strategies such as these are not helping, it might be time to consult a healthcare provider. You might be experiencing hyperacusis, a heightened sensitivity to normal environmental sounds, which can require professional treatment.

You might not be able to control the volume of the world around you, but you can control how you react to it. With the right techniques and tools, you can make your world a quieter, more peaceful place to be. Just remember, while sensitivity to noise can be annoying, it's just a phase, and like all phases, it has a volume knob. Here's to finding yours.

Increased Clumsiness

If you've been dropping things or stumbling more than usual, don't be too hard on yourself. It's not just 'one of those days;' it could very well be one of those perimenopausal symptoms.

The Causes

Hormones Playing Tricks: If you've suddenly become a magnet for mishaps, it's probably not a sudden loss of grace. Hormonal changes, particularly fluctuations in oestrogen, can affect your spatial awareness. That's right, those hormones are sneaky; not only do they mess with your temperature and mood, but they can also fiddle with your brain's GPS.

Stress: The Silent Saboteur: Stress can also heighten clumsiness. When you're stressed, your body goes into 'fight or flight' mode, which isn't particularly useful when you're just trying to walk across the room without tripping over the carpet.

Self-Help Strategies

Mindfulness: Take a moment to pay extra attention to your movements. If you find yourself frequently stumbling, a little mindfulness can go a long way. Instead of multi-tasking, try uni-tasking for a change. Give your full attention to each action, whether it's walking, lifting, or even just grabbing your coffee cup.

Keep Moving: Regular exercise can help you get back in touch with your body and improve your coordination. Think simple and effective, like yoga or Pilates. These exercises not only improve your flexibility but also focus on intentional movement, which can help you be more mindful of your body's position in space.

Home Safety: It's also worth looking at your environment. Are there any hazards like loose carpets, electrical cords, or scattered toys that could be contributing to your newfound clumsiness? A little home improvement might just prevent a lot of unnecessary spills.

A Nutritional Nudge: Believe it or not, certain nutrients like vitamin D can play a role in muscle function and stability. So, consider getting your levels checked, and if you're falling short, a supplement might just help you find your footing again.

Consult a Healthcare Provider: If you've tried all these steps and you're still feeling like a bull in a china shop, it might be time to consult a healthcare provider. There could be other underlying issues affecting your coordination or spatial awareness.

Increased clumsiness during perimenopause can feel like a comedy of errors, but you are certainly not alone, and more importantly, you're not doomed to a life of spills and thrills. With some mindful adjustments and a dash of self-compassion, you can regain your poise or, at the very least, get a good laugh out of the journey back to gracefulness.

Banging into Walls/Loss of Balance/Tripping

Are you navigating your own home like it's a labyrinth and you're the Minotaur? If you're bumping into walls, tripping over furniture, or just generally feeling off-kilter, don't worry – you're not transforming into a living, breathing pinball.

The Causes

Hormones Take the Stage, Again: Yes, you guessed it – those ever-changing hormones are back for an encore performance. This time they're messing with your vestibular system, which is responsible for your sense of balance and spatial awareness. It's like your internal gyroscope got a bit tipsy.

Stress: Besides hormones, stress can also throw your balance off. When stressed, your focus narrows, potentially making you less aware of your surroundings and thereby increasing your chance of an unintended collision course with walls or furniture.

Self-Help Strategies

Vestibular Rehabilitation: It's a bit like a balance boot-camp. Consider giving vestibular rehabilitation exercises a whirl as I suggested with vertigo too. These are targeted exercises that can help you get back that feeling of stability you might be missing. The focus is on improving balance, enhancing vision, and fostering mental clarity – all good things when your living room has suddenly turned into an obstacle course.

Mindfulness: Yes, I'm pulling the mindfulness card again, because it's really that useful. Being present in the moment isn't just great for your mental well-being; it's also key for not mistaking the living room wall for an open door. Take your time when moving from place to place, whether you're at home, at the office, or walking in the park.

Safety First: Check your home for "trip and bump" hazards. Loose rugs? Pin them down. Random clutter on the floor? Time to declutter. You might also consider installing some softer lighting, which can help you better gauge distances and reduce glare that might disorient you.

Footwear Matters: Believe it or not, the type of shoes you wear can impact your balance. Opt for comfortable, flat shoes with a good grip. That pair of high heels might look fabulous, but they're not doing you any favours if you're already feeling unsteady.

Consult a Healthcare Provider: If all else fails and you still feel like a sailboat in a storm, consult a healthcare provider. It could be an inner ear issue, a medication side effect, or some-thing else entirely.

Navigating your way through perimenopause might feel like you're in a never-ending game of 'don't touch the lava,' but with some mindful practices and the right advice, you'll be back to your nimble self in no time. Just remember, everyone's a little clumsy sometimes.

CHAPTER 23

The Perimenopausal Potpourri

Other physiological symptoms

If perimenopause were a film, it would be a multi-genre blockbuster featuring drama, action, mystery, and maybe even a little horror. From body odour changes to restless legs syndrome, the range of symptoms can be as varied as a British weather forecast. So, let's embark on this roller coaster ride of physiological symptoms, and don't worry, there are ways to make the journey smoother.

Body Odour Changes

If you've suddenly noticed that your personal fragrance has shifted from roses to something less pleasant, rest assured, you're not alone. While there are no specific UK statistics on this, anecdotal evidence suggests that changes in body odour are a common issue among perimenopausal women.

The Causes

Hormonal Havoc: Our dear old friend, the hormone oestrogen, is back in the spotlight. The hormonal shifts during perimenopause can turn your usual scent into something a bit... funkier. Oestrogen helps regulate your sweat glands, and when it goes on holiday, your scent can go a little haywire.

A Whirlwind of Factors: In addition to hormonal shifts, stress, diet, and certain medications can also play a role in your newfound scent. A diet rich in certain foods like garlic, onions, or spices can contribute to a more pungent aroma. Medications can also cause body odour as they metabolise and exit your body.

Self-Help Strategies

A Good Scrub: More frequent showers are your first line of defence. Your favourite (natural-as-possible) soap can further help because it targets the bacteria that mingle with sweat to cause odour – paying particular to underarms, at the top of your thighs and around your public area, and any other areas where sweat tends to accumulate.

Dietary Tweaks: What goes in must come out, and that includes through your sweat. Eating a balanced diet rich in fruits and vegetables can actually improve your scent. Avoiding foods known to cause odour, like asparagus or fish, might also be beneficial.

Natural Deodorants: Many women find that switching to natural deodorants can help. Look for ones that contain baking soda or arrowroot powder, as these natural ingredients can help absorb moisture and neutralise odour. See the back of this book for my recommendations.

Breathable Fabrics: Your choice of clothing can make a significant difference. Opt for natural, breathable fabrics like cotton, which allow your skin to breathe and can reduce sweat – and by extension, odour. Bamboo is my absolute fave as its thermoregulating too.

Consult a Healthcare Provider: If you've tried all of the above and you're still battling a stubborn stench, it might be time to consult a healthcare provider. There may be other under-lying issues that need to be addressed, from thyroid conditions to dietary intolerances.

Body odour changes during perimenopause are annoying but usually manageable. With some lifestyle tweaks you'll get back to smelling like your fabulous self in no time. After all, life's too short to spend it feeling – or smelling – less than wonderful.

Phantom Smells

Ever walked into a room and smelled freshly baked cookies, only to find no such thing in sight? Or maybe you've caught a whiff of something foul with no identifiable source? Welcome to the world of phantom smells, where your nose takes on a life of its own. Sadly, it's not a sign that you've developed superpowers – although, how cool would that be?

The Causes

Hormonal Hijinks: So, what's up with these mysterious, non-existent smells? No, your house is not haunted; your hormones are just playing tricks on you again. Oestrogen, that ever-fluctuating hormone, seems to have its fingers in yet another perimenopausal pie. It's a key player in how your olfactory system functions, and when it's in flux, your sense of smell can go on an emotional roller coaster too.

Your Brain on Scents: It's not just hormones; your brain can also play tricks on your nose. Stress, migraines, and even certain medications can trigger phantom smells. So, if you smell burnt toast but haven't burnt any, don't panic. It's probably not a psychic prediction of your future cooking fails.

Self-Help Strategies

Clear the Air (Literally): An air purifier can be a game-changer. While it won't stop phantom smells, it will ensure that your nose isn't picking up on real, albeit faint, odours that might be mistaken for imaginary ones. Plus, cleaner air is always a bonus.

Aromatic Distractions: A temporary solution could be to focus on real, pleasant scents. Light a lavender candle or diffuse some essential oils to ground your senses. However, be mindful about what you're using, as strong fragrances can sometimes exacerbate the issue, and the more natural, the better (see the section on xenoestrogens).

Mindfulness and Relaxation Techniques: Given that stress can sometimes trigger phantom smells, relaxation techniques such as deep breathing or mindfulness meditation could provide a respite. After all, a calm mind often leads to a less adventurous nose.

Consult a Healthcare Provider: If you find yourself plagued by persistent phantom smells, it might be time to see a healthcare provider. There could be a range of underlying issues, from sinus problems to neurological conditions, that may need to be ruled out.

Life might be handing you lemons – in scent form, at least – but you don't have to just sniff them and bear it. With a few strategies and perhaps a doctor's visit, you can get your olfactory system back on track.

Chest Pain

Chest pain can be the sort of thing that gets you frantically googling your symptoms, convinced you're seconds away from a serious medical event. And while it's absolutely crucial to rule out any life-threatening issues, it's worth knowing that you might just be experiencing another delightful feature of perimenopause.

First off, let's set the stage with some reassuring data. The NHS notes that many women in their perimenopausal years report experiencing chest pain that turns out not to be connected to heart disease. It's as if your body said, "What else can I throw into the mix to keep her on her toes?"

The Causes

Hormones Strike Again: Guess what? Hormones are the culprits once more. The ever-volatile oestrogen levels during perimenopause can impact your cardiovascular system, leading to a variety of symptoms, including chest pain. So, while it's tempting to think that your heart is sending you Morse code for 'SOS,' it's often more of a false alarm.

First Things First: Always Consult a Healthcare Provider: Before you brush off chest pain as just another quirk of perimenopause, it's vital to get it checked out by a healthcare provider. Heart issues are no joke, and you'll want to rule those out before doing anything else. Plus, you get to enjoy the thrill of EKG stickers and perhaps even a treadmill test. Think of it as a spa day, but for your internal organs.

Self-Help Strategies

Once you've got the all-clear from your doctor, there are several ways to manage these chesty sensations:

Deep Breathing: Simple deep breathing exercises can help relax the muscles around your chest and may alleviate minor discomfort.

Regular Exercise: Physical activity, particularly cardiovascular exercise, can help strengthen your heart and improve your overall well-being. Just consult with your healthcare provider about what level of exercise is appropriate for you.

Herbal Remedies: Some women swear by herbal teas like hawthorn, which is often used for heart health. However, consult your healthcare provider before trying any herbal remedies, especially if you're on other medications.

Diet: Foods rich in omega-3 fatty acids, like fish and flaxseeds, can support cardiovascular health. But, as ever, consult your healthcare provider for per-sonalised advice.

Stress Management: Techniques like mindfulness and meditation can help you focus and may reduce stress, which is always good for your heart.

Experiencing chest pain during perimenopause can be quite scary. But once you've ruled out any serious health concerns, try some of these strategies to manage this uncalled-for drama.

Shortness of Breath

When you find yourself huffing and puffing from merely pottering about the garden or going up a flight of stairs, you may think you're suddenly unfit and old aged (I know I did). But rest assured, you're not alone. Shortness of breath is frequently voiced by many women navigating the labyrinth of per-imenopause.

The Causes

Hormones: At this point in the book, I am well aware that I genuinely sounding like a broken record, but hormones truly do have their fingers in many pies, and the respiratory system is no exception. Fluctuating oestrogen levels during perimenopause can affect your breathing patterns, making even simple tasks feel like you've run a marathon – sans medal or finish-line photo, unfortunately.

Consult a Healthcare Provider: Before you start planning your oxygen bar-themed 50th birthday party, it's essential to consult a healthcare provider. Persistent or severe shortness of breath could indicate underlying issues, such as asthma or heart conditions, that require proper medical evaluation. No one wants to jump from perimenopause to hypochondria, but it's always better to be safe.

Self-Help Strategies

Once you've been given the green light that it's just another perimenopausal quirk, there are ways to manage your newfound lack of breath.

Breathing Exercises: Techniques like diaphragmatic breathing and the '4-7-8 technique' (inhale for four seconds, hold for seven, and exhale for eight) can help improve lung function and decrease shortness of breath. Think of it as yoga for your lungs – just with less stretching and no awkward poses.

Cardio Exercise: While you may feel like avoiding any extra panting, regular cardiovascular exercise can help improve your lung capacity. So, whether you're into swimming, walking, or dance aerobics, pick an activity that gets your heart rate up – but please consult your healthcare provider to tailor your exercise plan.

Hydration: Believe it or not, staying well-hydrated can help thin mucus in the airways, making it easier to breathe. So, guzzle down that H_2O like you're a contestant in a water-drinking challenge.

Natural Remedies: Some women find relief with herbal solutions like eucalyptus or pepper-mint oils, known for their respiratory benefits. However, always consult a healthcare provider before diving into the herbal world, especially if you're on medication for other conditions.

Shortness of breath is just one of those unexpected twists that makes you hold onto your hat (and your lungs) in perimenopause. With proper medical guidance and some proactive strategies, you'll be breathing easy and back to chasing after grandchildren – or just running upstairs without turning into a wheeze machine – in no time.

Breast Soreness/Tenderness

Just when you think you've ticked all the symptom boxes, your breasts decide to throw their hat into the ring. According to a UK study, up to a whopping 70% of women in perimenopause experience breast soreness or tenderness. That's 7 in 10 women who might feel like they're wearing an invisible 'Caution: Sensitive Area' sign across their chest.

The Causes

Hormones: As per usual, hormonal fluctuations are the leading ladies in this delicate drama. When your oestrogen and progesterone levels decide to stage their own version of 'Dancing on Ice,' the result can often be a change in breast tissue, making everything from hugs to tight tops a potential 'ouch' moment.

Immediate Action: Seek Professional Help: It's crucial to consult a healthcare provider if you find that your breast soreness is becoming a headline act in your life. Yes, it's easy to brush off the symptoms as just another perimenopausal quirk, but it's always better to exclude other potential issues. Breast soreness could be indicative of other health conditions or imbalances that require professional evaluation.

Self-Help Strategies

Supportive Bras: If your bras are more vintage than versatile, it might be time for an upgrade. Invest in a well-fitted, supportive bra, preferably one without underwire, as that can exacerbate soreness. Consider a sports bra for periods of heightened tenderness. A little support goes a long way – think of it as a hug your breasts won't shy away from. Or a bamboo shaper bra for a softer-than-soft, gentle lift.

Cold/Warm Compresses: Sometimes, good old temperature therapy can be a woman's best friend. A warm compress can help ease the pain, while a cold compress can reduce swelling. You're basically turning your freezer and kettle into a home spa for your breasts.

Natural Remedies: Evening primrose oil is often touted as a natural remedy for breast pain, as it's believed to balance hormone levels. Always consult a healthcare provider before adding any supplements to your regimen, especially if you're already on **other** medications.

Dietary Changes: Cutting back on caffeine and salt may also help alleviate symptoms. These two seem to aggravate breast tenderness in some women. It's almost like coffee and chips are joining forces against you, but it might be worth it to cut back and see if things improve.

Over-the-Counter Relief: Non-prescription anti-inflammatory medications like ibuprofen can provide short-term relief from breast soreness. But again, consult your healthcare provider for long-term solutions and to ensure it doesn't interact with any other medications you may be taking.

Breast soreness can make even the simplest activities – like hugging loved ones or sleeping on your stomach – a real challenge. But with proper medical advice and some practical lifestyle tweaks, you can minimise discomfort and continue leading a 'breast assured' life (apologies for the terrible pun!).

Breast Swelling

If you're dealing with this symptom, you're not alone. While there aren't specific UK statistics to back this up, the sheer volume of conversations and questions I have had indicate it's a pretty common experience during perimenopause.

What's causing your new 'balloon animals,' you ask? Well, as hormones like oestrogen and progesterone go on their hormonal merry-go-round, they can affect fluid retention in your body. The end result? Your breasts may swell, leaving you feeling like you've got water balloons rather than the usual flesh and blood.

If your bust decides to bust out and it becomes a persistent issue, don't just consider buying a bigger bra. Consult a healthcare provider for a thorough evaluation. While breast swelling during perimenopause is generally not a red flag for serious medical conditions, it's always good to rule out other potential causes.

Self-Help Strategies

Supportive Bras: No, we're not talking about a bra that listens to your problems, although that would be amazing. We're talking about well-fitted, supportive bras that can help alleviate the discomfort that comes with swelling. Look for options with wide straps and full coverage. Your boobs need a hug, not a squeeze!

Cold Compress: A good old-fashioned cold compress can offer some relief. The cold helps to reduce swelling and numb the area a bit. Just don't go overboard – you don't want frostbite on top of everything else.

Anti-Inflammatory Foods: Foods like turmeric, ginger, and omega-3-rich fish can help combat inflammation, potentially reducing swelling. But remember, no food is a miracle cure. Always consult your healthcare provider if symptoms persist.

Limit Salt and Caffeine: Too much salt can contribute to fluid retention, and caffeine can aggravate breast tenderness. Try to limit these in your diet and see if it makes a difference.

Natural Diuretics: Foods like asparagus, parsley, and beets are known for their diuretic properties, which can help with fluid retention. But again, consult your healthcare provider if you're thinking of making significant changes to your diet.

Hydration: It might seem counterintuitive to drink more water when you're retaining fluid, but staying hydrated can actually help your body release extra water.

Breast swelling is one of those symptoms that remind us of the joys of womanhood at every life stage. It might not be a barrel of laughs, but with some proactive measures, you can make it a little less bothersome.

Electric Shocks

You may feel like you've been turned into Buzz Lightyear or like a character in a science fiction movie, getting hit by invisible laser beams, but don't fret – you haven't been abducted by aliens. Some women going through perimenopause report sensations that feel like electric shocks. Although it's less common, affecting a smaller percentage of women, it's enough to make you jump, quite literally!

The Causes

What's causing this shocking turn of events? You guessed it – our hormonal friends are at it again. The ebb and flow of hormones like oestrogen during perimenopause can mess around with nerve function. These hormones usually keep our nerve and tissue functions in check, but when they decide to go on a roller coaster, things can get a bit, well, zappy.

Immediate Action: Call in the Experts

Experiencing electric shocks isn't just disconcerting – it's downright unsettling. So, if you find yourself repeatedly struck by these 'lightning bolts,' don't try to endure them alone. Consult a healthcare provider for a thorough evaluation and proper diagnosis. The sensations could be linked to other health issues that require medical attention. Better to zap the problem in the bud, so to speak.

Self-Help Strategies

Stay Hydrated: One of the simplest yet most effective tips. Staying well-hydrated can help maintain optimal nerve function and may alleviate the frequency of electric shocks. Aim for at least eight cups of water a day – think of this as an 'unplugging' strategy for your internal electrical system.

Balanced Diet: Sometimes, deficiencies in vitamins like B12 can exacerbate nerve issues. Make sure your diet is rich in essential nutrients to keep those nerves as stable as possible.

Mindfulness and Relaxation Techniques: Stress can aggravate your symptoms. Mindfulness, meditation, and relaxation techniques can help you stay grounded – pun intended – and may reduce the occurrence of electric shocks.

Exercise Regularly: Physical activity is known for its benefits on the nervous system. Regular exercise can help to improve nerve function and may reduce the severity or frequency of electric shocks. Just avoid exercises that themselves cause a jolt or shock to the system. No need for extra shock value!

Feeling like you're getting tiny electric shocks might not be your idea of a party trick, but with the right approach and medical advice, you can dial down the voltage on this peculiar symptom. So, here's to less buzzing and more smooth sailing through perimenopause!

Tingling Extremities

Tingling extremities, also known as 'pins and needles,' are a symptom that a fair number of perimenopausal women report.

So, what is the tingle behind the jingle? Well, hormonal changes that are the daily bread of perimenopause can influence nerve function. This could lead to that tingling or even numb sensation. If the tingling becomes a recurring symptom in your life, don't ignore it. Consult a healthcare provider for a thorough evaluation. While tingling extremities are usually benign, they could be a sign of other underlying issues, such as vitamin deficiencies or nerve conditions.

Self-Help Strategies

Regular Exercise: You don't need to train for a marathon, but some moderate exercise can improve circulation, potentially easing those tingles. Something as simple as a brisk thirty-minute walk daily can work wonders for your overall circulation.

Stretch It Out: Light stretching exercises can also boost circulation and may help relieve symptoms. Take frequent breaks if you're sitting or standing for extended periods and give those limbs a good stretch.

Hydrate: Sometimes, dehydration can lead to tingling sensations. Make sure you're drinking enough water, especially if you're also engaging in exercise.

Magnesium and Vitamin B Supplements: Some people find relief by taking magnesium or vitamin B supplements, which are known for their role in nerve function. However, consult your healthcare provider before starting any new supplement regimen and see the end of this book for more on supplements.

Warm Compress: A warm compress can also encourage blood flow and may help if the tingling is due to poor circulation. Just don't make it too hot – you don't want to go from tingling to tinged.

Mindfulness and Relaxation Techniques: Believe it or not, stress can make the tingling worse. Practices like mindfulness and deep-breathing exercises can help you relax, improving your overall well-being.

So, if your extremities are experiencing the tingles, know that it's a sensation shared by many. It may not warrant a high-five, but with some proactive self-care, you can at least ensure that those tingles aren't anything more than a perimenopausal quirk.

Allergies or Sensitivities

Ever find yourself sniffling around your favourite bouquet of flowers or sneezing when the cat strolls by – your own cat that you've had for years, mind you? While it might seem like your body is suddenly rejecting things it used to love, you're not alone. Many perimenopausal women find that their immune systems become a bit more temperamental during this phase.

The Causes

So, what's causing this sudden shift from tolerant to touchy? Blame it on hormonal changes affecting your immune system. The fluctuations in hormones like oestrogen can make you more susceptible to allergies or sensitivities. It's like your immune system is suddenly throwing a tantrum, saying, "I don't like it anymore!"

Consult a Healthcare Provider: Persistent sniffles and sneezes warrant a visit to your healthcare provider. They can conduct tests to identify whether you're genuinely developing new allergies or if something else is at play. A thorough evaluation is your first step toward a sniffle-free life.

Self-Help Strategies

Allergy Testing: Knowing is half the battle. Tests can identify what's suddenly causing your immune system to rebel so you can take steps to avoid those triggers.

Air Purifiers: If you find that you're allergic to dust or pet dander, investing in an air purifier can make a significant difference in your home environment.

Dietary Adjustments: Foods can also be a common culprit when it comes to allergies and sensitivities. A slight modification in your diet may help.

Always consult with your healthcare provider before making significant dietary changes, though.

Natural Remedies: Certain herbs like butterbur and stinging nettle have been reported to alleviate allergy symptoms. Similarly, a teaspoon of local honey a day could potentially help your body adapt to local allergens.

Over-the-Counter Antihistamines: For less severe allergies, over-the-counter antihistamines can offer temporary relief. But remember, these are not a long-term solution and should only be used after consulting with a healthcare provider if you need them for more than a few days.

Reducing Stress: Believe it or not, stress can exacerbate allergies. Relaxation techniques such as deep breathing and meditation can sometimes reduce symptoms.

So, if your immune system is becoming picky in your perimenopausal years, you're not alone. While it's an inconvenience, it's also a chance for a health check-up, a little home

improvement, and perhaps even a new hobby in relaxation techniques. And let's be honest, who doesn't need another reason to invest in self-care? Keep those tissues handy, but with the right approach, you might not need them for long!

Restless Legs Syndrome

Okay, let's get one thing straight: if your legs are suddenly jumpy, it's not because they're planning a solo adventure without you. Restless legs syndrome (RLS) is more common than you might think, affecting up to 10% of the UK population. And if you're a perimenopausal woman, the likelihood of experiencing this can be even higher.

The Causes

So why are your legs so restless? The hormone imbalance that accompanies perimenopause can shake things up in the leg department. But it's not just hormones; poor sleep and stress can also be backstage players in this restless leg gig.

Consult a Healthcare Provider: If you're experiencing consistent symptoms, a healthcare provider can offer a thorough evaluation and recommend treatment options tailored for you. This might include medications to manage the condition, so don't hesitate to consult an expert.

Self-Help Strategies

Regular Exercise: Physical activity, particularly when done in the morning, can help alleviate symptoms. However, try to avoid vigorous exercise close to bedtime as it can actually worsen symptoms.

Iron Supplements: Low levels of iron are often linked to RLS. Consider adding iron-rich foods like spinach and legumes to your diet, or take a supplement after consulting your healthcare provider.

Warm Baths and Massages: Warm baths and leg massages can relax your muscles and might just tell those restless legs to take a chill pill.

Avoid Stimulants: Caffeine, alcohol, and tobacco can exacerbate RLS symptoms. Limiting these can be beneficial.

Leg Elevation and Compression Stockings: Elevating your legs or wearing compression stockings during the day can improve blood flow and may alleviate symptoms.

Natural Remedies: Some people find relief from RLS symptoms through acupuncture and even yoga. It's all about what works for you, so it might be worth exploring these options.

Mindfulness and Relaxation Techniques: Sometimes, practicing mindfulness and other relaxation techniques can help calm both your mind and your legs.

Having restless legs can be a frustrating experience, but remember, you're not alone. In fact, think of it as an opportunity to focus on taking better care of yourself. After all, your legs might just be telling you they need a little TLC, and there's nothing wrong with that. So, whether it's a jog in the morning or a soothing bath in the evening, there are plenty of ways to quiet those dancing legs and find your own rhythm again.

Changes in Vision

So, you're squinting at your book or enlarging the text on your phone and you're thinking, "Blimey, am I getting old, or is this print getting smaller?" Before you start shopping for a magnifying glass, remember that changes in vision can be another chapter in the perimenopausal saga.

The Causes

Hormonal changes during perimenopause are the likely culprits messing with your perfect vision. These fluctuations can affect eye tissues and fluids, potentially leading to dry eyes, sensitivity, and changes in vision, including difficulty focusing on close objects. It's like your eyes decided to go through a midlife crisis along with the rest of you, but instead of buying a sports car, they're going for blurry vision.

According to various studies, vision changes are a widespread issue among perimenopausal women. And it's not just about reading – some women report difficulties in depth perception, making parking the car an exciting new challenge.

Consult a Healthcare Provider if persistent issues with your vision continue. A healthcare provider can offer a thorough examination and, if necessary, corrective solutions, which may include glasses, contacts, or even eye drops for dry eyes.

Self-Help Strategies

Regular Eye Exams: Regular check-ups can catch changes early and give your optometrist a chance to adjust your prescription if you already wear glasses or contacts.

Quality Lighting: Ensure you have good lighting when reading or doing close work. Some-times, it's not you; it's the room that's too dim!

Breaks and Exercises: If you're working in front of a screen for long periods, take breaks and practice some simple eye exercises to relieve strain.

Hydration and Nutrition: Drink enough water to keep those peepers moist and eat foods rich in vitamin A and omega-3 fatty acids for eye health.

Natural Remedies: Some people swear by bilberry extract for improving vision. However, always consult your healthcare provider before starting any new supplements.

Blue Light Glasses: If you spend a lot of time in front of a computer, you might want to invest in blue light blocking glasses to reduce eye strain.

Mindfulness Techniques: Although it won't cure blurry vision, mindful relaxation can help ease the strain that your eyes might be under.

While it might be a bit disconcerting to realise your vision isn't what it used to be, it's not the end of the world. On the contrary, it's an opportunity to focus (pun intended) on self-care. Whether it's upgrading your lighting at home, booking regular eye check-ups, or exploring natural remedies, there's a whole menu of ways to be proactive about your eye health. So, take it all in, blink a few times, and remember it's never too late to see things clearly.

Dry Eyes
If your eyes feel like they've taken up residence in the desert and you're battling dryness on a daily basis, join the club. It's not just the hot flushes; your eyes are going through the perimenopausal drama as well. While it can be irritating (literally), dry eyes are far from rare, especially during this life stage.

The Causes
Ah, those hormonal fluctuations. They seem to be the gift that keeps on giving, don't they? During perimenopause, changes in hormone levels can

have a big impact on tear production. Essentially, your eyes have decided that now is a good time for a drought, when you're already coping with other perimenopausal symptoms. Talk about bad timing.

Up to 30% of adults report experiencing dry eyes, and guess what? The rates are even higher among perimenopausal women. You can almost imagine your eyes joining a support group, can't you? "Hi, I'm an eyeball, and I'm dry."

Consult a Healthcare Provider for persistent dry eyes; it's always wise to get professional advice. Your healthcare provider might suggest diagnostic tests or treatments you haven't considered.

Self-Help Strategies
Artificial Tears: Over-the-counter artificial tears can be a quick fix for occasional dryness. But remember, not all artificial tears are created equal; some are better for specific issues like redness or allergy relief.

Humidifier: Adding moisture to your indoor air can help alleviate dry eyes. It might make your skin happy, too!

Natural Remedies: Omega-3 supplements have been shown to improve tear quality, making them a potential natural solution for dry eyes. However, consult your healthcare provider before starting any new supplements.

Eye-Friendly Diet: Foods rich in omega-3 fatty acids like salmon or chia seeds can contribute to eye health. Keep those eyes 'well-fed'!

Hydration: You've heard it a thousand times, but it's worth repeating – stay hydrated. Every part of your body, including your eyes, benefits from proper hydration.

Blink Exercise: It sounds silly, but conscious blinking can help refresh your eye's tear film. Try a 'blink break' every twenty minutes when doing close-up tasks or screen time.

Avoid Triggers: Windy conditions, smoky areas, and air-conditioning can worsen dry eyes. Try to minimise exposure when possible.

Warm Compress: A warm, wet cloth over your eyes for a few minutes can help stimulate tear production. Plus, it feels rather soothing.

While dry eyes might make you feel like you're living in a perpetual sand-storm, remember, you're not alone, and there are plenty of steps you can take to improve the situation. From natural remedies to high-tech humidi-fiers, the options are wide-ranging. Keep those eyes moist, and they'll thank you by letting you see the world a little clearer.

Increased Susceptibility to Infections

If you're wondering why you're suddenly catching every cold, sniffle, and flu in a fifty-mile radius, don't be too hard on yourself. No, you haven't become the neighbourhood germ magnet overnight. Believe it or not, many peri-menopausal women find themselves more prone to infections.

The Causes

The hormonal roller coaster can also wreak havoc on your immune system. Research suggests that oestrogen and progesterone play a role in immune function. As their levels fluctuate during perimenopause, your body's de-fence mechanisms might not be as robust as they once were.

While there aren't specific UK numbers focusing on perimenopausal women and infections, it's estimated that adults catch two to four colds a year on average. If you find you're exceeding that quota, it might not be sheer bad luck but rather the hormonal shifts that come with perimenopause.

Self-Help Strategies

Good Hygiene: Yes, it's not just something you nag your children about. Washing your hands frequently, avoiding close contact with sick individuals, and keeping surfaces clean can go a long way in keeping you infection-free.

Boost Your Immune System: Incorporate immune-boosting foods into your diet. Citrus fruits, garlic, and spinach are excellent choices. Some studies suggest that foods high in antioxidants can strengthen the immune system.

Stay Hydrated: Good old water flushes out toxins, and a well-hydrated body is better equipped to fight off infections.

Get Active: Moderate exercise can help boost your immune system. Even a thirty-minute walk a few times a week can make a difference.

Vitamin Supplements: Consider taking vitamin C or zinc supplements to bolster your immune system. However, do consult your healthcare provider for advice tailored to your needs. See more on supplements at the back of this book.

Sleep Well: A lack of sleep can weaken your immune system. Aim for seven to eight hours a night to keep your immune system in tip-top shape.

Herbal Remedies: Echinacea and elderberry are commonly used herbal remedies believed to boost immunity. But please, always consult with your healthcare provider before taking any new supplement.

Mindfulness and Stress Reduction: High stress levels can weaken your immune system. Consider mindfulness techniques or even short meditative sessions to lower stress levels.

Probiotics: A healthy gut can support a robust immune system. Consider adding a probiotic supplement to your daily regimen or eating probiotic-rich foods like Greek yoghurt.

Consult a Healthcare Provider: If you find yourself falling ill more frequently than an actor in a soap opera plot, it's time to consult a healthcare provider for a full evaluation and to discuss any other treatment options available to you.

Remember, when it comes to health, a bit of prevention is often better than a pound of cure. Take steps to boost your immune system and consult healthcare providers as needed, because perimenopause shouldn't feel like a never-ending flu season.

Changes in Sense of Taste

Finding that your favourite chocolate doesn't hit the spot like it used to? Before you write a strongly-worded letter to Cadbury, take a step back. You're not morphing into a fussy eater or an elite food blogger. Many perimenopausal women report changes in their sense of taste. So, if your palate's doing a flip, it could be hormonal.

The Causes

You probably have guessed why by now (sorry, for being a broken record) but oestrogen levels are all over the shop during perimenopause, and guess what? These hormones can affect the 10,000 taste buds that are nestled on your tongue. This can result in changes to how you perceive sweet, salty, sour, and bitter tastes. You're not just imagining it; your taste buds could be playing tricks on you.

This phenomenon is not a rarity. It's one of those under-discussed symptoms that can be frustratingly overlooked. A study published in the journal *Menopause* found that roughly 40% of the women reported experiencing a change in their sense of taste or smell during perimenopause.

I completely went off red meat and alcohol in the perimenopause. The thought of a juicy steak, which was once something I would love, has me been turning green now. Certain cheeses too are an absolute no-go (especially the stinky ones).

Self-Help Strategies

Stay Hydrated: Water is essential. Staying hydrated is crucial for optimal taste bud function, and it can also help in neutralising any weird flavours you might be experiencing.

Mindful Eating: Being more attentive when eating can sometimes recalibrate your taste buds, allowing you to enjoy your food more.

Spice It Up: Sometimes introducing new spices and flavours can stimulate your taste buds. From chilli to basil, experiment a bit. Who knows, you might discover a new favourite dish in the process!

Cut Down on Sugar and Salt: Changes in taste might mean you're overcompensating by adding extra sugar or salt. Try to use natural herbs and spices to season your food instead.

Zinc Supplements: Zinc plays a role in the maintenance of taste and smell. You could consider a supplement but consult your healthcare provider first.

Oral Health: Keep up with your dental hygiene. Sometimes, a lingering bad taste can be attributed to poor oral health.

Consult a Healthcare Provider: If you're considering auditioning for *MasterChef* just to figure out what's going on with your taste buds, it might be time to consult a healthcare professional for a thorough evaluation and to discuss treatment options.

Gargling and Rinsing: Sometimes a simple salt water rinse or using a mouthwash can freshen your mouth and temporarily reset your sense of taste.

Citrus Magic: Sometimes, citrus fruits like oranges and lemons can give a quick kick to your taste buds.

Second Opinions: Before you decide that your cooking has gone downhill, perhaps have a friend or family member taste your meals. It could be reassuring to know it's not your culinary skills but your taste buds that are off.

So, if you find that your beloved morning coffee suddenly tastes like dishwater, don't panic. Perimenopause might be the critic behind your changing taste reviews, but there are plenty of ways to coax those taste buds back into line.

THE UNCOMPLIKATED GUIDE TO PERIMENOPAUSE

Increased Sensitivity to Alcohol or Caffeine

A sip of wine suddenly feels like you've had the whole bottle, and a single cup of coffee sends your heart rate into overdrive? You're not just imagining it. You might just be joining the ranks of perimenopausal women who find that their tolerance for alcohol and caffeine has changed. Before you start thinking you've turned into a lightweight overnight, let's delve into why this happens and what you can do about it.

The Causes

Hormonal upheaval can affect liver function and the way your body processes substances like alcohol and caffeine. So, yes, your body isn't processing that glass of red or shot of espresso the way it used to.

A study published in the journal *Menopause* suggested that perimenopausal women might metabolise alcohol more slowly than they did in their younger years. Similarly, caffeine sensitivity has been observed to increase with age.

Self-Help Strategies

Moderation: As tempting as it is to have that second cup of coffee or an extra glass of wine, moderation is key. Try alternating with a glass of water or opting for herbal teas.

Timing Matters: If you're sensitive to caffeine, avoid consuming it in the afternoon or the evening. This could disrupt your sleep, leading to a cascade of other symptoms.

Opt for Decaf: Love coffee but can't handle the jitters? Decaf can be a good compromise. It allows you to enjoy the ritual without the overstimulation.

Hydrate: Alcohol and caffeine can dehydrate you. Drinking plenty of water can mitigate some of the effects.

Know Your Limits: Keep a diary of how different amounts of alcohol or caffeine affect you. This can help you establish new limits for yourself.

Eat Well: Having food in your stomach can slow down the absorption of alcohol and caffeine, making their effects less intense. Opt for nutrient-dense meals that are rich in protein and fibre.

Go Herbal: For those who enjoy a hot drink, herbal teas like chamomile or peppermint can be good alternatives that come without the caffeine punch.

Consult a Healthcare Provider: If you're finding that even small amounts of alcohol or caffeine are wreaking havoc on your system, it's wise to get a professional opinion. Your GP can rule out any other potential causes and discuss appropriate treatment options.

Get Moving: Exercise can sometimes help in metabolising alcohol and caffeine more efficiently. Even a short walk can make a difference.

Mindfulness and Relaxation: Sometimes, we reach for a drink or a coffee as a way to cope with stress. Stress-relief techniques like meditation or deep-breathing exercises could offer a healthier alternative.

Check Labels: Many over-the-counter medications contain caffeine, especially in cold or headache tablets. Be aware of what you're taking, especially if you're already feeling sensitive.

Remember, it's not about giving up your favourite drinks; it's about adapting and finding new ways to enjoy them without the unwelcome side effects. Your body is changing, and that's OK. You're not alone in this; we're all in the same hormonal boat, just trying to steer through perimenopause without spilling our decaf. Cheers!

Increased Tendency to Bruise

Have you've noticed that you're sporting more purple patches than a tie-dye tee-shirt? No, you haven't become an overnight klutz; you might just be experiencing what many perimenopausal women report – an increased tendency to bruise. Before you start donning bubble wrap, let's look at what's causing this rather colourful development and how to navigate it.

The Causes

Once upon a time, you could bump into a table and walk away unscathed. But now, your hormones are rearranging the furniture in the house that is your body, and your skin's taking the brunt. The hormonal shifts that come with perimenopause can affect the elasticity and thickness of your skin, making you more susceptible to bruises even from minor bumps.

One study in the *Archives of Dermatology* indicates that skin thickness decreases by about 6.4% for each postmenopausal decade, increasing your chances of bruising.

Self-Help Strategies

Good Nutrition: Consider bumping up foods rich in vitamin C, vitamin K, and zinc. These nutrients are essential for skin health and healing. Oranges, strawberries, and kiwi are good sources of vitamin C, while leafy greens can provide vitamin K.

Stay Hydrated: Keeping your skin hydrated will make it more resilient. Drink plenty of water and consider using a hydrating skin cream.

Mind Your Steps: While it's not always possible to avoid accidents, being conscious of your movements can help. Take it slow when you're in unfamiliar surroundings.

Protective Gear: If you're into sports or activities that could result in bruises, consider wearing protective gear. No, you don't have to go full knight-in-shining-armour, but padded sleeves or knee guards could help.

Arnica Cream: This homeopathic remedy is often cited for its ability to reduce bruising and swelling. It's available over the counter and can be applied to unbroken skin.

Avoid Sun Damage: Ultraviolet rays can weaken your skin over time. Always use sunscreen or wear protective clothing when you're out and about.

Ice It: If you do get a bruise, applying ice can reduce blood flow to the area and potentially minimise the bruise.

Warm Compress: After the initial swelling has gone down, a warm compress can help dissipate the blood that has pooled under the skin.

Consult a Healthcare Provider: If you're decorating your skin with bruises too easily, or if they take an unusually long time to heal, it's best to seek professional advice to rule out any other underlying issues.

Blood Thinners: If you're on medications that thin the blood, consult your healthcare provider. They might be contributing to your ease of bruising.

Moderate Alcohol: Excessive alcohol consumption can also thin the blood and make bruising more likely. Moderation is key.

So, while it might seem like your body is playing bumper cars, these little changes can go a long way in preventing the unsolicited artwork on your skin. After all, bruises should be earned in epic adventures, not from bumping into the coffee table. Stay fabulous and take care!

Restlessness

If you're tossing, you're turning, and you're pacing up and down the living room like you're waiting for exam results, you might be going through what many women experience during perimenopause: a sense of restlessness that makes it hard to sit still. Let's break down why this might be happening and how you can channel this extra energy for good.

The Causes

Fluctuating hormones, as we have discussed, can have a profound impact on your mood and sleep quality. Poor sleep can, in turn, contribute to daytime restlessness. It's a classic chicken-and-egg scenario but with hormones and insomnia as the key players.

According to the Sleep Council, about 40% of people in the UK suffer from some form of sleep issue at some stage in their life. With sleep being a major contributor to restlessness, it's safe to say the issue is more common than you think.

Self-Help Strategies

Relaxation Techniques: Deep breathing exercises, meditation, or progressive muscle relaxation can serve as mini vacations for your mind. And who doesn't like a good holiday, right?

Exercise: Physical activity, particularly aerobic exercise, has been shown to improve mood and sleep quality. Just try not to exercise too close to bedtime, or you'll wind yourself up rather than wind down.

Mindfulness and Grounding: Feeling restless can be like having your head in the clouds. Grounding exercises, like touching a piece of fabric or focusing on your breath, can help bring you back to earth.

Warm Baths: A warm bath before bed can relax your muscles and also provide a psychological boundary between your busy day and bedtime. Plus, who doesn't enjoy feeling like a pampered goddess?

Cut Down Stimulants: Keep an eye on your caffeine and alcohol intake. Both can interfere with sleep and contribute to restlessness. Maybe switch that late-afternoon espresso for an herbal tea?

Healthy Sleep Environment: Make your bedroom a sleep sanctuary. A dark, cool room with comfortable bedding can do wonders for your sleep quality.

Natural Aids: Some people swear by herbal remedies like valerian root or melatonin supplements for better sleep. However, consult a healthcare provider before starting any new supplement.

Set a Routine: Our bodies love routine. Try to go to bed and wake up at the same time every day. Even on weekends. Your body's internal clock will thank you.

Consult a Healthcare Provider: If your restlessness feels like a never-ending game of musical chairs, it might be time to seek professional help. They can rule out other potential causes and provide targeted treatment options.

Remember, you're not alone on this restless journey. Many are sailing in the same boat – or rather, pacing in the same room. Implementing some of these strategies can help you find your inner Zen or, at the very least, give you something constructive to do while you're up and about.

Navigating the complex landscape of perimenopausal symptoms can indeed be challenging, yet it's essential to remember that you're far from alone on this journey. There's a shared experience here, a common thread that binds women going through similar challenges. It's a phase of life that millions have traversed before you, and millions will traverse after you. The road might feel arduous at times, but with a dose of humour and the right coping strategies and support, this period can be more manageable than you might think.

Gathering information and seeking advice, either from healthcare providers or through self-help resources like this book, can offer not just solutions but also much-needed peace of mind. Whether it's fluctuating moods, changes in taste, or an unexplained restlessness, knowing what to expect and how to manage these symptoms can be empowering. Moreover, focusing on natural remedies, proper nutrition, and a balanced lifestyle can not only alleviate your symptoms but also offer a sense of control at a time when it feels like your body is running its own show without consulting you.

While perimenopause comes with its set of challenges, it's also an opportunity to understand your body better and to prioritise your well-being. In the grand scheme of things, perimenopause is just one chapter in the book of your life, albeit a pretty eventful one. This is a period that also offers the time to reflect, make necessary adjustments, and to take the reins on your health and happiness.

With the right guidance, resources, and perhaps even a supportive community (as I mentioned earlier, you are so welcome to join my support group on Facebook), managing perimenopausal symptoms is not only achievable but can also be enlightening. So, take each day as it comes, arm yourself with knowledge, and remember that this too shall pass. This phase of your life could very well be a stepping stone to a more enlightened, health-conscious, and even more fabulous you. After all, life doesn't pause for perimenopause, and neither should you.

Navigating the myriad symptoms of perimenopause can feel like you're walking through a maze blindfolded. But remember, you're not alone. With the right strategies and a bit of humour, you can get through this phase with your sanity intact. So, while perimenopause might feel like a physiological potpourri, it doesn't have to be a Pandora's box. With the right guidance and support, you can manage these symptoms and continue to live your life to the fullest.

CHAPTER 24

HRT Backstage Pass

A journey through hormone history

We've talked, a *lot*, about the myriad of symptoms of perimenopause, and the why and what of how it can all make you feel. So now for a bit of better news – the levels of healing and help you can go through/get to relieve those troublesome symptoms and preserve your future health.

Perimenopause is not a disease or an ailment, it is simply a new chapter. Why not yell, "Plot twist!" and understand that it is just different. The old you, the pre-perimenopause you, no longer exists and you can't go back to being 'her.' But . . . you can feel more like yourself, just a different, wiser, more experienced version of yourself. So, before you look at the healing levels below, or decide which road to take, please know that the road doesn't lead back to your old self, it leads to a transition, and at the end of that, the new you will emerge (who can be your favourite self *ever*!).

I'm guessing that for many of you, the main question would be whether or not to take HRT to help you. With scare stories rampant in the media about HRT, and then other women lauding it as their saving grace, which way do you go? What would I recommend?

To be super-clear, I cannot tell you what would be best for you and what to choose. But what I can do is give you all of the research, information, and feedback I have about HRT – as well as the other choices – then you can make the most informed decision that feels right for you. The opinions about HRT are polarising so you will never please anyone, so please don't try to; do what is best for your body.

Even for perimenopause itself, some will say that it's a natural process to go through and we should learn to embrace it; and others will say God must be a man, because no woman would make women suffer in this way after years and years of periods, pregnancy, PMT, and the like; and yet more will tell you to throw everything you can at it to make it all go away.

I think I fall somewhere in the middle, personally. It is natural, we do have to embrace it (we have no option in that), but there are things that you can do to help yourself and that is what I would love to give you the knowledge on.

Oh, and while we're on the topic of 'right for you,' please, please, please make this decision yourself for your own body. It would be fabulous to have an understanding partner, or a well-meaning mummy, to discuss this with, and by all means, get their input; but the ultimate decision lies with you and what feels right for your body.

I will try to be as balanced and neutral as I can be, regardless of my own personal journey, as this is for you to decide (with input from your important humans and your medical team).

For many obvious reasons, the first thing we would discuss is HRT. However, before we do that, I want to give you an historical view of HRT and the studies that pertain to it because it will help you to see why there was a 'scare' surrounding this topic. Time to debunk some myths!

The Glamour and Grit of Hormone Therapy: An Historical Voyage

Hormones have been the darlings of the medical field since the 1940s. Picture this: extracting progesterone at that time required the corpus lutea of a jaw-dropping 50,000 pigs. For a dash of testosterone, you'd have to sieve through 4,000 gallons of urine. Oh, and let's not forget that in 1941, progesterone came with an eye-watering price tag of $200 per gram. Yes, science has thankfully moved on, and you won't find any job adverts for that particular lab assistant role.

The Swinging '60s: Forever Young with a Pill?

Come the 1960s, and hormone therapy was practically a fashion statement among women. Dr Robert Wilson penned his best-selling book, *Feminine Forever*, branding perimenopause as a "totally preventable" hormone deficiency disease. The promised elixir of youth? Oestrogen. Though appealing, we would later discover that the tale wasn't so straightforward.

A Reality Check in the '70s: Everything in Balance

The 1970s served us a slice of humble pie with research indicating that using oestrogen without progesterone upped the risk of endometrial cancer. This led to the birth of combined hormone replacement therapy (HRT), blending synthetic progesterone (progestins) with oestrogen in tinier doses. Because let's face it, moderation is key.

The 1993 Milestone: The Women's Health Initiative

Fast-forward to the '90s, and in comes the Women's Health Initiative (WHI) – a study with the colossal budget of $1 billion. Its aim? To thoroughly examine healthcare strategies for post-menopausal women. This study is the reference manual that continues to influence medical opinions on hormone therapy. It involved 16,608 women, some receiving a cocktail of Premarin and Provera, while others were given a placebo. But come 2002, the show abruptly stopped. Headlines screamed about

HRT's links to a 26% increased risk of breast cancer, 29% of heart attacks, and a staggering 41% of strokes.

The Domino Effect: Unravelling the Panic

The impact was seismic. Prescriptions for HRT plunged by a precipitous 65-70% in that year alone. The fallout was substantial; a follow-up study by Kaiser Permanente in California discovered that some women had abandoned hormone therapy prematurely. Interestingly, the WHI study had shown that women who discontinued HRT were at a 55% higher risk of hip fractures.

Decoding the Data: Separating Fact from Fear

Still, the echo of WHI's findings reverberates today. It reported a 27% increase in breast cancer among women on HRT compared to those on a placebo. But Dr Avram Bluming and Dr Carol Tavris, the authors of *Oestrogen Matters*, clarified that this statistic "almost reached nominal significance" – or in plain English, it didn't. Thus, the perceived risk could be more smoke than fire. Updated data in 2006 even indicated no heightened risk of breast cancer, yet this news hardly broke the internet.

What Statistics Don't Capture

As of 2010, WHI authors revealed more deaths from breast cancer in the HRT group, but the numbers were far from alarming – 2.6 versus 1.3 deaths per 10,000 women. In statistical jargon, this was a wash, yet it didn't pacify public concern. So, while it's wise to assess the risks of any treatment, it's equally important to dissect the statistics and understand their nuances. After all, stats are like bikinis – what they reveal is suggestive, but what they conceal is vital.

A Twist in the Tale: The 2018 *Climacteric* Review

In the realm of scientific studies, not all is as it appears. A 2018 review published in the journal *Climacteric* turned some heads. It revealed that women who diligently took their oestrogen-only Premarin pills had a substantial 32% reduction in breast cancer rates compared to those on a placebo. Hold the phone! There was also a 29% drop in ductal carcinoma, the most common type of breast cancer. In terms of the grand scheme of life and death – across 7,489 deaths recorded during WHI's eighteen-year follow-up – those on oestrogen didn't show any increased risk of dying from cardiovascular issues or cancer. Yes, that's a chunky morsel of food for thought.

The Devil's in the Demographics: WHI's Achilles Heel?

One thing the WHI study didn't brag about was its participant demographics. Picture this: the average participant was 63 years old and had been postmenopausal for about twelve years. As Drs Avram Bluming and Carol Tavris noted, a significant portion of the women were either overweight (35%) or obese (34%). Nearly 36% were on high blood pressure medication, and almost half had a history of smoking. Talk about a red flag – multiple red flags! Only a meagre 10% of the women were aged between 50 and 59. Considering that obesity alone is a risk factor for cancer and heart diseases, these stats cast a long shadow over the study's conclusions.

The Long Shadow of WHI: Dispelling Old Ghosts

Even today, the WHI study continues to haunt perceptions about menopausal hormone therapy (HRT). With a sample size of 80,955 postmenopausal women, the study suggested that ceasing HRT led to a 55% higher risk of hip fractures. The WHI study is like that old schoolmate who shows up in your Facebook memories – you can't easily forget them, nor the impressions they have left.

Questioning the Gospel: The Revelations of 'Oestrogen Matters'

But hang on a minute: not everyone is singing from the WHI hymn sheet. Drs Avram Bluming and Carol Tavris presented a rather riveting counter-narrative in their 2018 book *Oestrogen Matters*. They argued that the WHI's claim of a 27% increase in breast cancer risk was, to put it bluntly, not up to scientific snuff. The infamous "almost" in statistical significance translates to "not significant" in everyday lingo. Moreover, updated 2006 findings further dented the WHI's credibility, though these new insights didn't quite make it to the cover of *OK! Magazine*.

So, there we have it – science is an ever-evolving field, and clinging to outdated information can do more harm than good. It's time to keep up with the times, folks!

The Million Women's Study: Another Tale

In 2003, the Million Women's Study (MWS) claimed that 20,000 new cases of breast cancer in the UK were due to HRT usage. But when analysed rigorously, this claim deflated to a 0.3% increase per 1,000 women per year – hardly a figure to set alarm bells ringing.

The Media Scare: A Grain of Salt, Please

In 2019, headlines asserted that the risk of breast cancer from HRT was double the prior estimates. This claim traced back to a review that amalgamated data from 58 studies conducted between 1992 and 2018. However, this melange of data included outdated HRT types and observational studies, where participants weren't assigned treatments randomly. Many findings were gleaned from the WHI and MWS, which, as we've established, have their limitations.

Assessing the Risks and Lifestyle Choices

Now, don't get me wrong: it's crucial to assess the risks of any medication. However, let's not lose sight of the fact that lifestyle choices, such as diet and alcohol consumption, also have significant roles to play. For example, it's estimated that 50% of breast cancer cases could be prevented by improving lifestyle choices.

According to Cancer Research UK, drinking more than fourteen units of alcohol a week is linked to a 20% increase in breast cancer risk. Yet we don't see the same uproar about wine as we do about HRT.

Inherited and Lifestyle Risk Factors

We cannot control some risk factors, such as family history or the age at which we experience perimenopause. However, smoking, heavy drinking, and being overweight are choices we can definitely rethink. And let's not forget the often-overlooked polycyclic aromatic hydro-carbons (PAHs) found in smoked foods and charred meats, which have been linked to cancer.

Know Your Body

Finally, regular breast and chest checks can't be stressed enough. In the UK, women between 50 and 70 are invited for mammogram screenings every three years. While screenings do save lives, around 4,000 women each year in the UK receive treatments they don't actually need. So, don't overlook the importance of being attuned to your own body.

In essence, it's time we approach the conversation around HRT and breast cancer with nuance rather than fear. Making lifestyle changes and staying informed can go a long way in reducing risks and improving quality of life.

CHAPTER 25

Level 1 of Healing

HRT

HRT can be very beneficial for people going through the perimenopause, and with the new type of transdermal HRT available, the benefits for many women far outweigh the risks (see the last chapter for more on this). As each of us wants to, and should, make our own choices on this topic, you'll need to know a bit about the different types of HRT and how they are used because, let's be honest, it's not a one-size-fits-all kind of deal. Think of oestrogen as the fertiliser and progesterone as the lawnmower, and you can see why they would need to be in balance with each other (to avoid an overgrown lawn).

Combined Hormone Therapy: The Balanced Act

This is like the bestie who brings out the best in you. It combines oestrogen with progestogen and it's ideal for women who still have their uterus. The addition of progestogen helps counterbalance the effects of oestrogen, reducing the risk of endometrial cancer. However, this isn't the go-to option for everyone; it can may carry some increased health risks, so it's crucial to have an open chat with your GP about it.

Cyclical Hormone Therapy: Timing Is Everything

Cyclical, or sequential, hormone therapy provides hormones in a cycle – oestrogen every day and progestogen for part of the month. This one mimics your natural menstrual cycle and is mainly recommended for women who are experiencing perimenopausal symptoms but are still menstruating. Think of it as syncing your internal clock with a trusted timekeeper.

Continuous Hormone Therapy: The Steady Companion

This is the no-fuss, consistent friend that you can always count on. You take both oestrogen and progestogen every day, which means there are no breaks, no menstrual-like bleeding, and – hooray! – potentially fewer mood swings. It is generally recommended for postmenopausal women who've said their final goodbyes to their periods completely.

Systemic Hormone Therapy: The Whole Shebang

This method is like treating yourself to a full spa day, not just a mani-pedi. Systemic therapies include pills, patches, and injections that impact your entire system. They're great for addressing a range of perimenopausal symptoms like hot flushes and night sweats. However, the spa day analogy isn't complete without mentioning that systemic hormone therapy is associated with higher risks, including blood clots and certain cancers.

Topical Hormone Therapy: The Local Hero

Topical therapies include creams, gels, and patches. These focus on specific areas and are the 'neighbourhood heroes' of hormone therapy. They're excellent for combating vaginal dryness and similar localised symptoms. But remember, they are not designed to address systemic issues.

Decoding the Hormone Replacement Puzzle

Hormone replacement therapy (HRT) is a subject that can be as overwhelming as trying to find a matching pair of socks in a laundry basket, especially if you're journeying through perimenopause. Let's simplify things by focusing on body identical transdermal HRT.

The Dynamic Duo: Oestrogen and Progesterone

Firstly, let's introduce the stars of the show: oestrogen and natural micronised progesterone. Oestrogen can make its grand entrance in the form of a gel, patch, or spray applied to the skin. Progesterone? It can be swallowed as a tablet or worn in a patch alongside oestrogen or be provided by the Mirena Coil. Choices, choices!

Timing is Everything: When to Take Progesterone

Next up, let's talk timing. If you're still marking periods on your calendar, progesterone is taken on days 14 to 28 of your cycle. If your periods have ceased, you'll take it continuously but at a lower dose. Remember, progesterone tends to make you drowsy, so it's best taken in the evening.

Side Effects and Alternatives: Managing Low Mood

Progesterone can affect your mood like a poorly-timed joke at a dinner party. If you find it's bringing you down, there's a workaround. Progesterone can be inserted vaginally so it stays localised, keeping your digestive system – and perhaps your mood – out of the equation.

All-Natural Ingredients: The Plant-Based Source

Now, where do these hormone heroes hail from? They're plant-based, sourced from yams. Imagine it as a farm-to-table experience for your hormones, if you will.

The Science Bit: Safety and Risks

Time for some data! According to a study in *The Lancet*, transdermal HRT formulations are linked to lower risks of blood clots. The clot risk here? Virtually zero. As for cancer, body-identical hormones have been shown to carry a lower risk than synthetic versions, although it's vital to get tailored advice from a healthcare provider.

Good News on Cost: It used to be that every single component of your HRT prescription in the UK would cost a full prescription price (currently – in 2023 – it's £9.65) which could add up and make it difficult for some women to pay for.

However, they have now brought an HRT PPC (HRT Prescription Payment Certificate) which is a one-off payment of £19.30 for 12 months (the cost of two single items). The HRT PPC covers an unlimited number of certain HRT medicines for 12 months, regardless of why they are prescribed. But as the HRT PPC does not cover all HRT medicines, it's best to check before paying in advance for one.

Body identical transdermal HRT is like the comfortable, sensible pair of shoes in the confusing world of menopausal treatment: practical, low-risk, and designed to make life a little bit easier. But, as with any treatment plan, always consult your healthcare provider to tailor it to your unique needs. It's your body, your hormones, and ultimately, your choice!

Examples of Brand Names in the UK:

Body Identical Oestrogens:

- Oestrogel – Gel
- Oestrodose – Gel
- Sandrena – Gel
- Evorel – Patch
- Estrodot – Patch
- Lenzetto – Spray

Progesterone:
- Utrogestan – Tablet (Body Identical)
- Mirena Coil (see more on this on the next page/s).

Synthetic HRT – The Pioneering Ancestor

Synthetic hormone replacement therapy could be considered the pioneer in the HRT world, having been around long before its body-identical or bio-identical cousins took to the stage. But what exactly is synthetic HRT, and how does it measure up to more recent formulations? Buckle up, as we embark on a journey through the often-misunderstood terrain of synthetic hormones.

Molecular Mismatch: Not Identical, But Effective

First things first: synthetic HRT is not identical to the hormones naturally produced by the human body. But that doesn't mean it's ineffective. It was the go-to option for many years, easing the symptoms of perimenopause for countless women. The caveat is that because it's not an exact match to natural hormones, the body might respond to it differently, affecting everything from efficacy to side effects.

Types of Synthetic HRT: The Animal Connection

Here comes the part that might raise eyebrows: some synthetic HRT, such as conjugated equine oestrogen (also known as Premarin), is derived from concentrated pregnant mares' urine. Yes, you read that right – horses' urine. The point here is that *synthetic* can sometimes mean *animal-derived*, which can be a turn-off for some people, especially if you're going for an all-natural approach.

The Efficacy Debate: How Well Does It Work?

When it comes to easing symptoms like hot flushes, night sweats, and mood swings, synthetic HRT has been shown to be effective. According to a 2017 study in *The New England Journal of Medicine*, synthetic HRT reduced the frequency of these symptoms by about 37%. However, it's not a one-size-fits-all solution, and some women find that the side effects outweigh the benefits.

The Risks: What You Should Know

Research has indicated that synthetic HRT, particularly in older formulations, may have a higher risk profile compared to other types. The study that I mentioned before by the Women's Health Initiative pointed to increased risks of blood clots, stroke, and certain types of cancer. However, it's worth mentioning that newer formulations and delivery methods have been developed to mitigate these risks.

Side Effects: A Mixed Bag

Some common side effects include nausea, headaches, and even breast tenderness. These are usually temporary and often subside as the body adjusts to the treatment. However, if you're someone who prefers to avoid any 'horseplay' in your medical treatments, these side effects, coupled with the animal-derived nature of some synthetic HRTs, might be a deterrent.

The Cost Factor: The Wallet Equation

Synthetic HRT tends to be more affordable than its bio-identical or body-identical counterparts. This price point can make it an attractive option for many, especially those without the luxury of choice. It's like opting for a reliable family car over a flashy but expensive sports car: it gets the job done without burning a hole in your pocket.

An Ongoing Evolution: Where Are We Now?

Medical science is ever evolving, and synthetic HRT is no exception. New formulations and delivery methods are continually being researched to reduce risks and enhance efficacy. So, while synthetic HRT might seem like yesterday's news, it's still a key player on the hormone therapy stage.

Conclusion: Synthetic HRT – A Considered, but Outdated, Choice

At the end of the day, synthetic HRT has its pros and cons. It's effective, widely researched, and generally more affordable. However, it's not-so-natural origins and potential side effects can be sticking points for some. The takeaway here is that it's crucial to consult your healthcare provider to find out whether synthetic HRT is the right fit for you. After all, when it comes to hormonal health, the aim is to hit the bullseye, not to shoot arrows in the dark.

Laboratory derived Oestrogens.

Combination Tablets
- Elleste Duet Conti
- Kliofem
- Kliovance
- Femoston Conti
- Indivina
- Premise
- Novofem
- Tridestra
- Trisequens
- Femoston

Combination Patches
- Evorel Conti
- FemSeven Conti
- Evorel Sequi
- FemSeven Sequi

The Mirena Coil – Your Intrauterine Sidekick

When it comes to managing perimenopause or hormonal imbalances, the Mirena coil has often been hailed as the unsung hero of the progesterone world. If hormone replacement therapy (HRT) were a theatre production, think of the Mirena coil as a backstage manager – often unseen, but critically important. Let's dive into why this little device has become the talk of the gynaecological town.

The Science: Levonorgestrel, the Progesterone Sub

The Mirena coil employs levonorgestrel, a synthetic form of progesterone, delivered directly to where it's needed most – the uterus. Why the uterus, you ask? Because direct delivery minimises systemic side effects. It's like having your cake and eating it, but without the additional calorie concerns.

A Godsend for Heavy Bleeding: Therapeutic Uses

One of the most lauded uses for the Mirena coil is in treating heavy menstrual bleeding. Studies indicate that Mirena reduces menstrual blood loss by 71-95%, which, let's be honest, could be a game-changer for many women. If your monthly cycle feels like a horror film set, the Mirena coil might just be your director's cut.

Longevity and Convenience: Set It and (Almost) Forget It

The Mirena coil isn't just a quick fling; it's more of a long-term relationship. Lasting up to five years, it offers a degree of convenience that pills or patches struggle to match. It's the crockpot of the hormone world: set it, forget it, and let it do its work while you go about your busy life.

Side Effects and Considerations: Every Rose Has its Thorn

Of course, no treatment is perfect (if only!). Some women may experience side effects such as spotting, irregular periods, or hormonal imbalances. However, these tend to be minor and often resolve over time. It's essential to discuss any concerns with your healthcare provider to ensure the Mirena coil is most compatible match. Think of it as a medical matchmaking service!

Safety First: A Low-Dose Strategy

One of the attractive features of the Mirena coil is its low-dose approach. Unlike systemic HRT, which circulates hormones throughout your body, the Mirena coil releases a small amount of levonorgestrel directly into the uterus. This localised approach has been associated with fewer systemic side effects, according to research published in the journal *Contraception*.

The Mirena, with its targeted delivery and long-lasting nature, offers an alternative for women who need progesterone but want to avoid the systemic approach of traditional HRT. Whether you're grappling with heavy bleeding or looking for an efficient, long-term hormonal solution, this device might just be your ticket to smoother sailing. However, as always, your personal medical history and needs should guide your treatment choices, so don't skip that essential chat with your healthcare provider. After all, in matters of health, one size never fits all!

Bio-identical HRT

One option that's been raising eyebrows and curiosity is bio-identical HRT. Unlike its body identical counterpart, this form of HRT isn't officially endorsed by regulatory bodies. Let's break down what it is, and why it's a subject of debate.

Legality and Regulation: Not a Seal of Approval

First things first: bio-identical HRT is not endorsed by key institutions like the British Menopause Society or NICE. While body identical HRT has been thoroughly researched and standardised, bio-identicals occupy a kind of 'wild west' space in the hormone world. They're obtained through a private doctor and concocted in small pharmacies, which means they're a bit like the artisanal, boutique option of the HRT market. The catch? They're unregulated and often expensive.

Personalisation: A Blessing and a Curse

These hormones are compounded based on individual blood or saliva tests, making them as unique as your fingerprint – at least for the moment. The pitfall? Our hormone levels fluctuate faster than fashion trends, making that perfect dose potentially obsolete before you know it. This leads to issues of efficacy and batch consistency, making it akin to a custom-tailored dress that suddenly doesn't fit any more.

The Role of DHEA: A Wild Card Element

Bio-identical HRT often includes DHEA, which is considered to be a precursor to oestrogen and progesterone. While the notion of a 'precursor' sounds promising (like a prequel to a blockbuster movie), the reality isn't as straightforward. The way each person converts DHEA can vary widely, making dosage management a game of hormonal roulette. Furthermore, the scientific literature doesn't offer much support for DHEA's effectiveness.

The Data Gap: What the Research Says (or Doesn't Say)

Although anecdotal reports about the benefits of bio-identical HRT abound, the hard science is scant. A report by the Endocrine Society warns against the use of custom-compounded hormones due to a lack of evidence on safety and effectiveness. Additionally, because these hormones are not standardised, they have not undergone the rigorous testing that more conventional treatments have. This leaves a gap in data large enough to drive a truck through.

Cost Factor: The Price of Customisation

The words 'private doctor' and 'small pharmacy' already hint at the price tag attached to bio-identical HRT. Besides being unregulated, these treatments can be costly, making them less accessible for a broad audience.

Conclusion: Proceed with Caution

Bio-identical HRT is like the mysterious, alluring guest at the dinner party: intriguing but somewhat elusive. While the idea of customised treatment sounds enticing, the lack of regulation, inconsistent efficacy, and the hefty price tag make it a path to tread carefully. As always, consult your healthcare provider for advice tailored to your unique needs. After all, when it comes to your health, you deserve nothing less than the full picture.

The 'T' in HRT – A Closer Look at Testosterone Replacement

When we look at hormone replacement therapy (HRT), oestrogen and progesterone typically steal the limelight. However, let's not overlook the supporting actor in this hormonal drama – testosterone. Yes, it's not just for the gents; ladies need it too! But how does it fit into the HRT puzzle, especially in the context of the UK's medical landscape? Let's roll up our sleeves and dive in.

Why Testosterone? The Unsung Hormone Hero

So, why might some women need testosterone? First off, testosterone isn't just the 'muscle and libido' hormone; it's more versatile than a Swiss Army knife. For instance, it has been found to play a role in cognitive performance and energy levels. According to the *International Journal of Women's Health*, insufficient testosterone levels may contribute to 'brain fog' and decreased cognitive agility. So, it's not just about what happens between the sheets, it's also about what's going on between the ears.

Available Options: The 'His and Hers' Debate

In the UK, the commonly prescribed testosterone replacement for women comes in a one-size-fits-all 'male form,' often available under the name Tostran. Many GPs are apprehensive about prescribing this version, given that its formulation is primarily designed for men. On the other side of the spectrum is AndroFemme, specifically crafted to suit the female physiology. However, it's only available privately, which limits its accessibility. Activists are pushing for its NHS approval, turning this into something of a hormonal justice campaign.

The Libido Factor: More Than Just a Flicker

One of the main reasons why women consider testosterone replacement is a noticeable drop in sexual desire and responsiveness. According to a study in the *Journal of Sexual Medicine*, about 32% of women experience low sexual desire, and about 8-12% find it distressing enough to seek treatment. With testosterone's role in enhancing libido, it's no wonder women are keen to explore this avenue. It's like trying to reignite the spark in a long-term relationship, but in this case, it's with oneself.

Caution! Don't Go Overboard: Androgen Dominance

While testosterone can offer numerous benefits, moderation is key. You definitely don't want to tip the scale into androgen dominance. Symptoms to watch out for include male pattern baldness, deepening of the voice, unwanted facial hair, and even poly-cystic ovaries. It's like adding a pinch of salt to enhance a dish: you don't want to pour in the whole salt shaker!

The Gender Gap: The Campaign for Female-Specific Formulations

One of the most significant hurdles in testosterone replacement therapy for women is the lack of female-specific formulations. Many people advocate for a more nuanced approach that acknowledges gender differences in hormonal needs. The campaign to make AndroFemme available on prescription is part of this broader narrative.

Economic Considerations: The Cost of Feeling Good

Testosterone treatments are not typically inexpensive. For example, the cost of AndroFemme can be a barrier for many, and its private-only availability often makes it unattainable for those who cannot afford it. The economic dimensions of accessing effective testosterone therapy underscore the importance of policy change to include female-specific formulations in the NHS portfolio.

The Future Outlook: Where Do We Go from Here?

Research into the efficacy and safety of testosterone replacement for women is ongoing. The conversation around making female-specific formulations, such as AndroFemme, available on prescription in the UK is gaining momentum. As our understanding evolves, the hope is that accessibility and options will too.

Striking the Right Balance

Testosterone replacement therapy can be a boon for women, from boosting cognitive functions to reigniting that dormant libido. However, navigating the UK's medical landscape can make you feel like you're walking through a maze blindfolded. We're in a period of flux, and things are shifting, albeit slowly. The key takeaway? If you're considering testosterone replacement, consult your healthcare provider for a balanced perspective tailored to your individual needs. After all, when it comes to hormones, it's all about finding that Goldilocks zone – just right, not too little, not too much.

A Spotlight on Localised Oestrogen

Vaginal health often takes a back seat in conversations about perimenopause and ageing. But let's face it, when the going gets tough – or should we say, dry – localised oestrogen can come to the rescue. Especially for women experiencing vaginal atrophy, this option provides a way to maintain intimacy without the associated pain and discomfort. Ready to delve into the details? Strap in!

What is Vaginal Atrophy? Understanding the Culprit

Vaginal atrophy is the less-talked-about, often-overlooked cousin of hot flushes and mood swings (go back to vaginal atrophy under *perimenopause symptoms* for more explanation). It involves thinning, dryness, and a loss of elasticity in the vaginal walls. According to a study published in *The Journal of Clinical Endocrinology and Metabolism*, about 50% of post-menopausal women experience symptoms of vaginal atrophy. However, only 20-25% seek medical advice, often due to the taboo around discussing such issues. The condition not only affects one's sex life but can become a real emotional hurdle for couples.

(See also the previous chapter on this topic.)

The Solution: Enter Localised Oestrogen

A range of products provide a small dose of oestrogen that works its magic right where it's needed: in the vagina. Unlike systemic HRT, this approach keeps the hormone confined to its area of application. Thus, it's not roaming around your body like an uninvited guest at a party, but rather sticking to its designated seat.

Efficacy: Does It Really Work?

According to a systematic review published in *The Cochrane Database of Systematic Reviews*, local oestrogen treatment effectively alleviates symptoms of vaginal atrophy. Women in the studies reported fewer instances of dryness, improved elasticity, and an enhanced sexual experience post-treatment. So, in short, it's not just a placebo; it's a proven method for making things better down there.

Safety: Can Everyone Use It?

Because it's a local application, the risk factors are significantly lower than systemic HRT. In fact, even some breast cancer patients may be able to use localised oestrogen therapy, though this is *always* a decision to be made in consultation with healthcare providers. According to the National Institute for Health and Care Excellence, localised oestrogen is a viable treatment option for those who have contraindications for systemic hormone replacement.

The How-To: Application and Types

Localised oestrogen comes in various forms: creams, tablets, and even rings that release the hormone slowly over time. These are typically applied directly into the vagina, making them a sort of 'targeted treatment' for vaginal atrophy.

Couple Dynamics: The Emotional Component

The emotional toll of vaginal atrophy often goes unspoken. The inability to engage in sexual activities can be isolating and drive a wedge between partners. While localised oestrogen can't solve the emotional aspects entirely, by relieving physical symptoms it can provide a pathway for couples to regain some of the closeness they may have lost. See also chapter 17 on relationships.

Availability: Where Can You Get It?

You can get localised oestrogen products via a prescription from your GP or from specialised healthcare providers. There's a range of options available, making it more likely that you'll find something to fit your specific needs and comfort level. You don't have to traverse the Amazon jungle to find it; a quick trip to the doctor should suffice.

Localised oestrogen presents an excellent solution for women grappling with the often-painful symptoms of vaginal atrophy. While it's not a one-size-fits-all miracle cure, it offers an effective, low-risk option for symptom relief. So, if you find yourself in the difficult terrain of vaginal atrophy, consider talking to your healthcare provider about localised oestrogen. There's no need to suffer in silence – or dryness**Testing**
You do not need a blood test to be prescribed HRT. HRT is prescribed based on your age and your symptoms. That said, people who are experiencing perimenopause symptoms and who are under 45 should get a blood test.

Please see chapter 5 for more information and guidelines.

The Clock is Ticking, or Is It?

When it comes to hormone replacement therapy (HRT), timing isn't just about setting your alarm clock to remember your next dose. It's about knowing when to start, what the benefits and risks are as you age, and how long you can keep going.

The Ideal Window: Perimenopause and Under 60

Ever heard the saying, "The early bird catches the worm"? Well, in the case of HRT, the early bird might just catch some hormonal balance! According to the National Institute for Health and Care Excellence, the ideal time to initiate HRT is during perimenopause or under the age of 60. The reason? Younger tissues are generally more receptive to hormonal fluctuations, making the transition smoother.

Statistics and Risks: The Numbers Game

As you age, the risks associated with HRT do slightly increase. For instance, a 2021 review in the *British Journal of Obstetrics and Gynaecology* states that women over 60 who are on HRT have a marginally elevated risk of developing cardiovascular issues compared to those under 60. However, it's crucial to keep in mind that the baseline risk is generally low to begin with. It's not a cliff, more like a gentle hill, but it's worth discussing with your healthcare provider to make an informed choice.

Longevity on HRT: A Lifetime Affair?

The body-identical form of HRT isn't like a summer fling; it's more of a long-term relationship. NICE guidelines suggest that as long as the patient is benefiting from the treatment, there's no fixed 'expiry date' for discontinuing it. So, if you're still reaping rewards like improved mood, better sleep, and easier-to-manage menopausal symptoms, it might be a case of 'HRT and me: together forever!'

The 'Over 60s' Dilemma: Better Late Than Never?

It's a common misconception that there is a strict 'sell-by date' for starting HRT. While younger might be better in terms of risk and overall effectiveness, it doesn't mean that you're out of options if you're over 60. However, if that is the case, the approach is generally more conservative, involving regular check-ups and potentially lower doses. But hey, if 60 is the new 40, then you've got plenty of time, right?

Why Timing Matters: The Benefits

Timing isn't just about avoiding risks; it's also about maximising the benefits. Early initiation during perimenopause can often lead to better control over menopausal symptoms like hot flushes, according to a study in *Menopause International*. It's almost like getting in on the ground floor of an exclusive club – the earlier you join, the more you get to enjoy the amenities!

Medical Monitoring: Keeping an Eye on the Clock

Even if you are taking body-identical HRT over the long haul, regular medical check-ups are essential. Think of it as your car's MOT, but for your body. Routine visits ensure that you're still getting the most out of the treatment and that any potential side effects are caught early.

The Takeaway: Your Personalised Timeline

Remember, while general guidelines are useful, your journey with HRT is unique. A one-on-one discussion with your healthcare provider will give you the tailored advice that's right for you. You're not just another statistic; you're a woman with individual needs, so make sure your HRT plan reflects that.

Conclusion: Time's Up! Or Is It?

When it comes to HRT, the early bird might get the worm, but the latecomers still have a chance at a full garden. With proper guidance, timing, and regular health check-ups, HRT can be a beneficial part of your life for years to come. So, go ahead, make that appointment and take time by the . . . ovaries? Either way, make sure you're making the most of what HRT has to offer you.

HRT Fears

Many GPs are still very cautious about prescribing HRT because perimenopause training is not mandatory, and many just do not have the knowledge or skills to feel confident in prescribing it. Many people are still worried about HRT because of the highly spun and premature results published by the Women's Health Initiative which showed a very conservative indication of a link between HRT (the synthetic type) and breast cancer. Please see the previous section on the History of Hormones for more on this.

CHAPTER 26

Stand Up and Be Counted

Your doctor's visits: your rights, your questions, and beyond

S o, if you've decided it's time to take the plunge and ask your GP about hormone replacement therapy (HRT). Kudos! This is a big step, and preparation can make the difference between leaving the appointment empowered, or discouraged. Here's your comprehensive guide on how to make that GP visit a grand slam, whether you're in the UK or the US.

UK Chapter: Hormones and How to Handle Your GP
Find a Sympathetic Ear: The Right Medical Professional

Firstly, be your own best advocate. When making the appointment, don't just settle for any available doctor. Ask the receptionist to direct you to a 'perimenopause-savvy' doctor or advanced nurse practitioner, or the member of the surgery that has had the latest menopause/perimenopause training. In the UK, only 24% of women feel that their healthcare providers are very well informed about perimenopause, according to a study published in the journal *Menopause* in 2019. So, make sure you're not part of that majority left in the lurch!

Double Up: Time is of the Essence
This isn't a rush job, so if you think you'll need more time to discuss your symptoms, ask for a double appointment. A bit of waiting now might save you months of unnecessary discomfort later.

Show and Tell: Your Symptom Diary
A list of your physical symptoms can be a compelling exhibit A. The Balance App or a good old-fashioned diary can help you track your symptoms for at least three months. Trust me, 'data' is the new magic word in healthcare. I highly recommend my free symptom tracker on www.myperimenopausesymptoms.com or the one in "*The Uncom-pliKated Perimenopause Journal*".

Period Report: The Monthly Breakdown
When it comes to your periods, detail matters. Are they as unpredictable as a British summer, or as regular as Big Ben? Light, heavy, irregular, spotting, clots, painful – put it all down. The more your GP knows, the better they can help.

Shared Responsibility: Two Heads Are Better Than One
Remember, your GP isn't a mind reader, nor a miracle worker. Mention that you're open to non-pharmaceutical options as well. Your willingness to explore different avenues could lead to a more personalised treatment plan.

Challenge The Misconceptions: Advocate for Yourself
Unfortunately, there are still GPs who think you need to be a certain age to be in perimenopause, or that you can't possibly be experiencing perimenopause if you don't have hot flushes. If your GP tells you any of these old wives' tales, ask for a second opinion. A survey by the British Menopause Society found that one in four women visiting a healthcare

provider about their perimenopausal symptoms felt that the clinician was unsympathetic. Don't settle for less!

Private Avenue: Last Resort

If you've hit a wall, don't worry. There's still the option of finding a private doctor through the British Menopause Society. Get your initial HRT prescription privately, and then switch to the NHS for ongoing treatment.

US Chapter: Crossing the Pond for Your Hormones

Picking the Right Doc: The American Way

Similar to the UK, not all healthcare providers in the United States are perimenopause experts. The North American Menopause Society has a useful search tool to find a certified practitioner near you.

The Insurance Maze: Be Prepared

Health insurance in the US can be complicated. Before your appointment, check whether your insurance covers your preferred treatment. A study in the *Journal of Women's Health* showed that cost is a significant barrier for 40% of American women seeking HRT.

Prescription and Coverage: The American Twist

Unlike the NHS, your insurance might require you to visit a specialist for your HRT prescription. Check whether a primary care doctor's prescription will suffice or if you'll need a referral.

Over-The-Counter: An American Phenomenon

The US has a variety of over-the-counter menopausal symptom relief options. While these don't replace a healthcare provider's advice, it's good to be aware of what's available.

Your Rights: Informed Consent and Choice

In the USA, you have the right to be informed about all available treatments. This includes discussing the risks and benefits, something mandated by Federal and State informed consent laws.

Asking for HRT, A Universal Language

Whether you're in the UK or the USA, the process of getting on HRT involves some common steps be informed, be prepared, and be your own advocate. Your age, your symptoms, and your individual needs should guide your treatment plan. So go ahead and make that doctor's appointment. Time to take control of your hormones and show them who's boss!

So, armed with this knowledge, have that heart-to-heart with your doctor or other healthcare professional to find your perfect hormone therapy match. Because every woman's experience with perimenopause is as unique as she is, and you deserve a therapy that understands *you*!

As with my own personal experience, it may take a few attempts to get the right fit for you, so trial and error may be the way to go. But as long as you know what the ins and outs are of each type of hormone and application, you can feel more comfortable being flexible.

Standards, Perimenopause/Menopause and Why You Should Care

The British Menopause Society (BMS) has thrown down the gauntlet with its new Menopause Practice Standards for Health Care Professionals that they release in July 2022. It's their way of saying, "All right folks, let's get our act together when it comes to treating perimenopause!" But before you dive into the PDF, let me break down what these standards mean for you, the healthcare professionals involved, and why they are so super important. I have written the link in the extra resources section at the back of this book and published it as a file in my Facebook support group.

The Importance of These Standards: Setting the Bar High

Let's put it this way: you wouldn't want to fly with an airline that doesn't adhere to strict safety standards, right? The same logic applies to healthcare, especially when it comes to something as nuanced and impactful as perimenopause. Perimenopause affects approximately 13 million women in the UK at any given time, according to the BMS. But despite the high numbers, there's often a disappointing lack of understanding and consistency in care. These standards aim to ensure that every healthcare provider dealing with perimenopause is on the same high-quality page.

What the Standards Cover: More Than Just Hot Flushes

The new guidelines offer a comprehensive approach, covering everything from diagnosis and treatment to the management of side-effects and ongoing care. They include various treatments like hormone replacement therapy (HRT), cognitive behavioural therapy (CBT), and even lifestyle changes. It's not just a one-size-fits-all document; it's more like a tailored suit that covers all possible scenarios.

The Nitty-Gritty: Key Points in the Standards
Diagnosis and Initial Assessment

The standards emphasise a symptom-led approach, which means you shouldn't have to go through unnecessary tests. They note that blood tests should not be used to diagnose perimenopause or menopause in women aged over 45.

Treatment Options

A plethora of treatment options are described, from HRT to non-hormonal medicines and lifestyle changes. Did you know that over half of the women who experience perimenopause symptoms never receive treatment? According to the BMS, these guidelines aim to bring that percentage down significantly.

Risks and Benefits

Healthcare professionals are advised to provide a balanced overview of the risks and benefits of each treatment option. Remember, every silver lining has a cloud, but the guide insists that you should know about both.

Follow-Up Care

Continuity is king, or queen, in this case! The standards recommend regular reviews, especially in the first three months of starting a new treatment.

For Healthcare Professionals: Brushing Up on Perimenopause 101

If you're a healthcare professional, consider these standards your new study guide. The National Institute for Health and Care Excellence (NICE) found that 71% of women seeking help for perimenopausal symptoms had to visit their healthcare provider more than once to get the help that they needed. These standards aim to change that by ensuring that the first visit is productive and informative.

For the Public: Empowerment through Knowledge

Arming yourself with these standards before heading off to see your GP can make a significant difference. It provides a framework for what you should expect in terms of care and treatment. So go ahead, give that PDF a quick read; it's essentially your cheat sheet for a better perimenopause experience.

The Bottom Line: Transforming the Future of Perimenopause Care

What the British Menopause Society has done here is not just raise the bar but set a new standard (quite literally!) for how perimenopause should be treated and managed. If followed diligently, these standards have the potential to revolutionise the experience of perimenopause for women in the UK.

So next time you're at the GP, perhaps nudge them (gently, of course) and ask if they're up to date with the new Menopause Practice Standards. After all, knowledge is power, especially when it comes to navigating the labyrinth that is perimenopause.

Non-Hormonal Drug for Hot Flushes

The Hot Topic of Hot Flushes

As I mentioned earlier, hot flushes are like those uninvited party guests who arrive at the most inconvenient moments and then refuse to leave. When you're going through perimenopause, these flushes can become frequent, unpredictable, and yes, quite bothersome. But hang on to your (cooling) hats because there's a new non-hormonal drug being tested that could be a game-changer!

The Science: Molecules and Pathways (Oh My!)

This promising development revolves around a molecule called NT-814. For those of us who aren't lab coat-wearing scientists, it's easy to think, "What is a molecule going to do for my hot flushes?" Well, NT-814 blocks neurokinin B and its sidekick, the neurokinin 3 R pathway. Imagine them as little traffic police saying, "Stop right there, vasomotor symptoms!" This pathway can go into overdrive when your oestrogen levels drop, leading to those dreaded hot flushes.

What is Vasomotor, Anyway?

The term 'vasomotor' refers to the dilation and constriction of blood vessels. When these functions are disrupted – thank you, declining oestrogen – you end up with hot flushes. Think of it as your body's thermostat going haywire. See more in chapter 21.

Statistically Speaking: Why This Matters

According to a study in the *Menopause* journal, approximately 75% of perimenopausal women experience hot flushes. Another survey found that almost a third of women rate their symptoms as moderate to severe. So, any new development in tackling this widespread issue is sure to make waves.

How it Compares to HRT

Hormone replacement therapy (HRT) is one of the most popular treatments for perimenopausal symptoms, but it comes with its own set of potential risks and side effects.

A non-hormonal drug like NT-814 could offer an alternative, without having to sacrifice efficacy.

The Waiting Game: Trials and Approvals

Even though NT-814 sounds promising, it's still going through clinical trials. In the fast-paced world of medical research, this is the equivalent of waiting for your nail polish to dry – it can't be rushed. Once it passes all the checks and balances, this new drug could be a significant step forward in non-hormonal treatments for perimenopause symptoms.

Why You Should Keep an Eye on This

In a nutshell, NT-814 has the potential to provide relief from one of the most common and irritating symptoms of perimenopause without resorting to hormonal treatment. For the countless women who either can't take HRT for medical reasons or prefer not to, this could be big news.

In Summary: A Glimmer of Hope in a Hot Situation

The development and testing of NT-814 could revolutionise the way we approach perimenopause and its notorious side-effects. While NT-814 is still in the trial phase, early signs point to a future where you might be able to attend a party without worrying about your uninvited hot flushes crashing the scene. Keep this one on your radar, ladies; it might just be the cool breeze you've been waiting for.

CHAPTER 27

Healing Level 2

Lifestyle

Perimenopause is full of ups, downs, and a few surprising twists. But fear not, because you have more control over this ride than you might think. Lifestyle changes can significantly influence your body's handling of blood sugar, stress levels, and thyroid function and more.

Control Freaks Rejoice: The CANs and CAN'Ts

Let's face it; we all like to have some level of control in our lives. Perimenopause may feel like an uncontrollable shift, but you can take the reins in several ways:

Things You CAN Control

- **Diet Choices**: Yes, what you eat and drink is within your domain. Choosing foods that regulate your blood sugar can aid hormonal balance.

- **Exercise Routine**: Movement can make a difference. Exercise can help regulate blood sugar and ease stress, but make sure you're not overdoing it, as excessive exercise can exacerbate hormonal imbalances.

- **Sleep Patterns**: Your bed is more than just a comfy place; it's your sanctuary for hormone regulation. Getting quality sleep helps balance your cortisol levels and reduces stress.

- **Mental Outlook**: Your perspective on life and its challenges has a more significant impact than you may realise. A positive outlook can influence your body's stress response.

- **Information Diet**: What you read, watch, or listen to can either stress you out or calm your nerves. Be mindful of the media you consume.

Things You CAN'T Control

- **Others' Opinions**: As much as you'd like to, you can't control what other people think or say.

- **Life's Curveballs**: Some things are just out of your hands, but you can control your reaction to them.

Environmental Awareness: Inside and Out

The term 'optimal environment' may sound like a fancy room with mood lighting and plush carpets, but it actually refers to an internal and external state where your body can function at its best. This environment allows your body to efficiently process hormones, balance blood sugar, eliminate waste, and adapt to stress.

Data Dive: Why Lifestyle Matters

A study published in *Menopause Review* indicates that lifestyle interventions like diet and exercise have a positive impact on the quality of life for perimenopausal women. Likewise, the American Psychological Association states that managing stress is crucial for overall health, especially during perimenopause.

Emotional and Mental Wellbeing: The Forgotten Frontiers

Let's not underestimate the power of emotional and mental health. Take this time as an opportunity to focus on yourself. It's not selfish; it's self-care. Besides, you can't pour from an empty cup!

Breaking the Cycle: No More Crutches

You know those daily crutches we rely on to get through stressful times? Perhaps it's that extra glass of wine or mindless scrolling through social media. Now's the time to break that cycle. Instead, why not pick up a new hobby or reconnect with an old one?

Your Life, Your Rules

Perimenopause may feel like constant change, but you have the power to set the house rules. By adopting the right lifestyle changes, you'll be better equipped to handle whatever this transitional phase throws at you. Remember, you can't control everything, but you can control enough to make a difference.

Nourishing Your Way Through Perimenopause

The perimenopausal transition is like your body's way of saying, "All right, we need to have a chat about how you're fuelling me these days." It's not just about cutting calories or following fad diets; it's about achieving a balanced and nutritionally dense way of eating.

Focus on Balance: The New Dietary Mantra

Forget counting every calorie as if it was a precious gem. During perimenopause, what is more important is the quality of what you're eating. The focus is on giving your body the nutrition it needs to manage stress, maintain hormonal balance, and yes, have the energy for movement.

Data Speaks: Diet's Influence on Perimenopause Symptoms

Studies have shown that women who follow balanced diets rich in essential nutrients have fewer perimenopausal symptoms. A study from the journal *Menopause* indicates that the Mediterranean diet significantly reduces hot flushes and night sweats. See below.

Mediterranean Magic: A Diet for the Ages

The Mediterranean diet shines like a culinary superstar when it comes to managing perimenopause. Rich in fresh fish, extra virgin olive oil, salads, fruits, and vegetables, it's like sending your body on a Greek holiday without the expensive plane ticket.

Why It Works

Not only is this diet high in essential nutrients and antioxidants, but it also includes lean proteins and healthy fats that help balance hormones and keep you feeling full and energised.

The Keto Question: A Temporary Fix?

Ketogenic diets are tempting for quick weight loss, but use them with caution. Prolonged use of high-fat Keto diets has been linked to increased cardiovascular risk. Always consult a health-care provider when considering this option.

Time-Managed Eating: Intermittent Fasting

Intermittent fasting is like giving your digestive system a 'Do Not Disturb' sign for a few hours. It offers your body a break, letting it focus on other vital functions like hormonal balance and cellular repair.

Caution on the Clock

However, going to bed hungry is like inviting a cortisol party into your body – something you don't want during perimenopause. Always consult with a healthcare provider before beginning intermittent fasting.

Low-Fat Diets: The Hormonal Faux Pas

Contrary to the popular diet culture, low-fat diets are not your friends during perimenopause. Hormones start their journey in cholesterol, so skimping on essential fats could backfire.

Sugar, Alcohol, Dairy, and Gluten: The Conditional Companions

Let's be clear: none of these are inherently evil, but moderation is key. Excessive consumption of sugar and dairy (cheese, we're looking at you) can wreak havoc on your hormonal balance.

Medicinal Uses: The Lesser-Known Heroes

Sugar can sometimes act as a 'first-aid kit' for shock, and a glass of wine might help you unwind after a particularly stressful day. However, always consider natural alternatives like breathing exercises and other holistic practices first.

Phytoestrogens: Your Plant-Based Allies
Understanding Phytoestrogens

Phytoestrogens, the versatile compounds found in plants, mimic the function of oestrogen in the human body. They can attach themselves to oestrogen receptors and help balance your hormonal landscape.

Here's where legumes, alliums, seeds, fruits, and vegetables come in. These foods are rich in phytoestrogens, compounds that act like a less potent form of oestrogen in your body. But, before you jump on the phytoestrogen train, ensure your liver and gut functions are in top shape.

Anti-Xenoestrogen Role

Interestingly, they can also block xenoestrogens which are the sneaky synthetic or natural compounds that mimic the hormone oestrogen. They are found in various products, including plastics, personal care items, and industrial solvents – potentially disrupting the delicate hormone balance and leading to oestrogen dominance.

It's as if these plant compounds are pulling double duty as security guards for your hormone balance.

I have personally created a whole lifestyle brand, originally stocked full of products that can help you in your perimenopause journey such as chemical free cleaning, beauty and bathing products, as well as bamboo bedding, nightwear and underwear as well. If you would like to take a look, you can go to www.kategrosvenorlifestyle.com.

Foods Rich in Phytoestrogens
- **Legumes**: Lentils, chickpeas, kidney beans and peas are not just for your grandma's stews anymore.

- **Alliums**: Think garlic, onions, and leeks. They not only add flavour to your meals but also some oestrogenic balance.

- **Seeds**: Flaxseeds are the star here, but chia and sunflower seeds make good supporting acts.

- **Fruits**: Apples, plums, and cherries make for a delicious, hormone-friendly snack.

- **Vegetables**: Time to give broccoli, carrots, and celery the respect they deserve!

- **Soybeans**: Love them or loathe them, soy products such as tofu can also offer a phytoestrogen boost.

Supplements and Professional Guidance
While it's wonderful to aim for a balanced diet rich in these foods, some people may still need a phytoestrogen boost through over-the-counter supplements or tinctures. It's crucial to consult an herbalist or nutritional therapist to get the dosage just right.

When to Proceed with Caution
If you're dealing with symptoms of oestrogen dominance, ensure your liver and gut function are in good shape before you invite phytoestrogens to the party.

Essential Fats: More Than Just a Culinary Trend
The Importance of Fats
Fats play a starring role in hormone production, beginning with choles-terol. So, when it comes to perimenopause, low-fat diets don't get an invite to the soirée.

Symptoms of Essential Fat Deficiency
Lack of essential fats can manifest in unpleasant ways, including depres-sion, joint pain, and those pesky sleepless nights.

Where to Find Essential Fats
- **Oily Fish**: Think salmon, mackerel, and sardines.
- **Nuts and Seeds**: Almonds and walnuts are excellent choices.
- **Egg Yolk**: Yes, the yolk, not just the white!
- **Extra Virgin Olive Oil**: A Mediterranean diet staple.
- **Tahini**: For when you need a break from hummus.

Recommended Supplements
See the section towards the back of this book on supplements that you can take to help you on your perimenopause journey and/or consult your healthcare provider about adding some.

Fibre: The Unsung Hero of Perimenopause
Why Fibre is Crucial
Soluble and insoluble fibre are essential for hormone regulation and a healthy bowel. Around perimenopause, they become the unsung heroes keeping your internal systems running smoothly.

Food Sources
Whole Grains:
Oats: Oats are rich in soluble fibre, which helps lower cholesterol levels. Brown Rice: Unlike white rice, brown rice retains the bran and germ layers, making it a good source of fibre.

Legumes:
Lentils: These are loaded with both soluble and insoluble fibre.
Chickpeas: Excellent for fibre and a good source of plant-based protein.
Black Beans: High in fibre and a great addition to various dishes.

Fruits:
Apples: A classic source of fibre, with both soluble and insoluble types.

Berries: Options like strawberries, raspberries, and blackberries are fibre-rich and packed with antioxidants.
Pears: Known for their high fibre content, especially in the skin.

Vegetables:
Broccoli: High in fibre and packed with vitamins and minerals.
Carrots: Not only rich in fibre but also a great source of beta-carotene.
Spinach: A leafy green with good fibre content and other essential nutrients.

Nuts and Seeds:
Chia Seeds: These tiny seeds are packed with fibre, especially soluble fibre that forms a gel-like consistency.
Almonds: A good source of both fibre and healthy fats.
Flaxseeds: Rich in fibre, omega-3 fatty acids, and lignans.

Whole Grain Pasta and Bread: Opt for whole grain versions for more fibre compared to their refined counterparts.
Cereals: Look for cereals that are labelled as high in fibre and low in added sugars.
Popcorn: Surprisingly, air-popped popcorn is a whole grain and a good source of fibre.
Quinoa: A versatile grain that's not only high in fibre but also a complete protein source.
Psyllium Husk: Often used as a dietary supplement, it's extremely high in soluble fibre and can help with constipation.

The Magic of Flaxseeds: A Triple Whammy

According to a study, flaxseeds are a powerhouse containing 75 to 800 times more lignans than other plant foods. Lignans are oestrogen-like molecules with cardio-protective and anti-inflammatory properties.

What's in a Flaxseed?

- **Omega-3 Fats**: For your brain and heart health.
- **Phytoestrogens**: Remember our plant-based allies?
- **Soluble and Insoluble Fibre**: For your digestive bliss.

How to Use Flaxseeds

You can have one or two tablespoons of ground flaxseeds per day. Soak them overnight for an easy-to-digest morning treat, or simply toss them into your salads, breakfasts, and soups.

Understanding the importance of phytoestrogens, essential fats, fibre, and the marvel that is flaxseeds can transform your perimenopausal experience. Always consult a healthcare provider for tailored advice. Here's to happy eating and a balanced perimenopause!

The Ultimate Guide to Simplifying Meal Prep: Featuring the Slow Cooker and More

Ah, Britain, the land of endless tea, drizzly weather, and the delightful queue. Amidst the hustle and bustle of UK life, meal prep can be the unsung hero that keeps us going. Here are my top tips on making meal prep a cinch, with a special nod to the British penchant for slow cookers (which I'm sure other nations love equally!).

Planning: Your Passport to Culinary Success

According to a YouGov poll, 12% of Brits are in the habit of eating the same lunch every single day. While there's comfort in consistency, a well-planned meal menu can inject some variety into your life and ensure a balanced intake of nutrients.

How to Get Your Plan Sorted

1. Identify what your diet is lacking – more protein, less sugar, etc.

2. Browse British go-to websites like BBC Good Food for inspiration.

3. Map out your weekly menu. Throw in a 'wild card' meal for when you want to indulge.

Bulk Buying: Economical and Eco-Friendly

Mintel reports that while 87% of British online grocery shoppers still physically visit super-markets, the appeal of online shopping is on the rise.

Top Tips for Bulk Buying

- Utilise apps like Ocado, Amazon Fresh, or Waitrose for grocery deliveries.

- Buy pantry essentials like rice and pasta in bulk to save money and cut down on waste.

Pre-Chopped Veg: The Time-Saver You Never Knew You Needed

Research from the University of Cambridge indicates that making veggies more convenient can significantly increase their consumption.

Storage Wisdom

- Use airtight containers and store your pre-cut veggies in the fridge for up to three days.

- For a longer lifespan, consider blanching your vegetables and stowing them in the freezer.

Keeping It Simple: A Less-is-More Approach

Sometimes the best meals are the simplest. And let's be honest, not every dinner needs to be a full Sunday roast.

Simplicity Resources

- Websites like BBC Good Food have a 'Quick and Easy' section for straightforward yet tasty recipes.

- Tesco also have a great easy recipe selection on their website.

Any recipes that I found great for perimenopause I have shared in my support group.

The Mighty Slow Cooker

Here's where the slow cooker takes centre stage. According to the charity Electrical Safety First, 57% of UK residents are proud owners of a slow cooker.

Why We Love Slow Cookers

- They're great for tenderising cheaper cuts of meat.

- Nutrients are better retained compared to some fast-cooking methods.

- Perfect for classic British fare like stews, casseroles, and even puddings.

Slow Cooker Tips

- Plan meals where you can throw in all the ingredients in the morning, and come home to a warm, ready meal.

- Choose recipes that align with your dietary goals – there are plenty of healthy slow cooker recipes out there.

Meal Box Services: The Modern Pantry

Meal box services like Hello Fresh and Mindful Chef are on the rise, with Statista predicting the market to grow to $2.44 bn by 2027.

Pros and Cons

- **Pros:** Convenient and often nutritionally balanced.

- **Cons:** Can be more expensive than DIY meals. Check for sustainability credentials before subscribing.

Whether you're in the Scottish Highlands, in a New York penthouse, or the heart of the countryside, meal prep is evolving into a critical part of daily life. It's not just about making a quick sandwich; it's about crafting a sustainable, balanced, and hassle-free approach to feeding yourself.

CHAPTER 28

Healing Level 3

Mental Health

Navigating the seas of perimenopause can sometimes feel like sailing through a storm – choppy waters, strong winds, and yes, the occasional bout of seasickness in the form of mental health challenges. As we embark on this chapter, we'll set our sights on the often under-discussed yet immensely important topic of mental health issues that arise during perimenopause. From the more commonly talked-about conditions like anxiety and depression to less discussed but equally significant issues such as feeling dead inside and emotional vulnerability, we'll delve into what you may encounter and how to find calmer waters.

It's important to remember that mental health isn't a side note in your perimenopausal journey; it's an integral part of the whole picture. Even if you've been a paragon of emotional equilibrium all your life, perimenopause can throw you a few curveballs. Fortunately, knowledge is power, and there are various ways to address and manage these mental shifts effectively. By the end of this chapter (and the next one on mindset too), you'll be armed with practical advice, resources, and perhaps most importantly, the reassurance that you're not alone on this journey.

Anxiety

Anxiety during perimenopause can feel you don't recognise your own thought processes anymore. While anxiety is not exclusive to this life stage, the hormonal changes happening in your body can turn it up several notches. A survey by the Nuffield Department of Population Health at the University of Oxford found that 22% of women aged 45-64 experience anxiety symptoms regularly. Moreover, NHS statistics indicate that one in six people in England report experiencing symptoms of anxiety or depression in any given week. When you throw hormonal imbalances like those occurring during perimenopause into the mix, you're dealing with a cocktail of factors that can seriously rattle your mental well-being.

One of the primary culprits for heightened anxiety during perimenopause is fluctuating levels of oestrogen. This hormone plays a crucial role in regulating mood by influencing the production and uptake of serotonin, often called the 'feel-good hormone.' When oestrogen levels are inconsistent, it can lead to mood swings and exacerbate feelings of anxiety.

Another contributing factor could be sleep disruption, which is common during perimenopause. Poor sleep quality has a direct link to increased anxiety levels, according to research published in the *Journal of Behaviour Therapy and Experimental Psychiatry*. Lack of sleep can make it harder to cope with stress, leading to a vicious cycle where anxiety further disrupts your sleep pattern.

Self-Help Strategies

Mindfulness: This is a potent tool for combatting anxiety. Multiple studies, including one published in *JAMA Internal Medicine*, have shown that mindfulness meditation can significantly improve anxiety symptoms. It doesn't have to be a thirty-minute session; even five minutes of focused breathing can make a difference. Sit in a comfortable position, inhale deeply through your nose, hold it for a few seconds, and then exhale through your mouth. Doing this repeatedly can help you feel more anchored and present, lowering your anxiety levels.

Cognitive behavioural therapy (CBT): Another highly effective treatment for anxiety. There are numerous CBT courses available online, tailored to varying degrees of anxiety. These courses help you identify triggering thoughts and replace them with more balanced and rational perspectives. They equip you with the tools you need to manage not just your current symptoms but also future bouts of anxiety. A meta-analysis published in the *Psychological Bulletin* found that CBT is particularly effective for treating anxiety and mood disorders, showing long-term benefits as well. See *"The UncompliKated Perimenopause Workbook"* for more on this.

Exercise is another option to consider. Physical activity releases endorphins, which act as natural mood lifters. Even moderate exercise can have a significant impact on reducing anxiety levels.

Nutrition is often overlooked but can be a crucial part of managing anxiety. For instance, a study in the *Journal of Clinical Psychology* found that foods rich in omega-3 fatty acids could reduce symptoms of anxiety. Adding more fatty fish, flaxseeds, and walnuts to your diet might help.

Lastly, if you find your anxiety symptoms overwhelming, don't hesitate to seek professional help. Sometimes medication like SSRIs (selective serotonin reuptake inhibitors) can provide the extra help you need in coping with anxiety.

Understanding that anxiety during perimenopause is a common experience can be comforting. But it's crucial to take proactive steps to manage it effectively. From mindfulness and CBT to exercise and nutrition, there are multiple paths you can take to reclaim your peace of mind.

Depression

Depression during perimenopause can feel like a huge weight is sitting on your chest, squashing the oxygen out of you. According to the Office for National Statistics, one in four women between the ages of 45 and 54 experience symptoms of depression, highlighting just how prevalent this issue is among women in this age group. It's not just about feeling down or having the 'blues;' perimenopausal depression is a complex interaction of hormonal changes, life circumstances, and mental health factors that can make life incredibly challenging.

One of the biological factors at play is the fluctuation in oestrogen levels. Oestrogen helps regulate mood by affecting the production of neurotransmitters like serotonin. When these hormone levels oscillate, it can throw your mental well-being off balance, leading to symptoms of depression. A study in the *Journal of Clinical Psychiatry* found that oestrogen therapy could be an effective treatment for perimenopausal depression, pointing to the critical role of hormonal fluctuations.

Another contributing factor could be sleep disturbances. Research published in *Sleep Medicine Reviews* found that poor sleep quality is linked to depression. During perimenopause, sleep problems like insomnia are frequent due to night sweats and temperature fluctuations. This can set up a vicious cycle, where lack of sleep exacerbates depression, and depression, in turn, disrupts sleep.

Life changes can also be a key factor. This stage of life often brings with it significant transitions such as children leaving home, career changes, or even retirement. These shifts can lead to feelings of emptiness or loss of purpose, fuelling symptoms of depression.

Self-Help Strategies

Exercise: it's not just good for your body; it's like a natural antidepressant. A comprehensive meta-analysis has shown that regular exercise can significantly alleviate symptoms of depression. You don't need to turn into a fitness fanatic overnight. Just twenty to thirty minutes of moderate exercise, like a brisk Weight or a simple home workout, can do wonders. The release of endorphins during physical activity serves as a mood booster, and the benefits can last for several hours post-exercise.

Seek support: Never underestimate the power of a strong support network. During this challenging time, isolating yourself is the last thing you want to do. A study in the *Journal of Abnormal Psychology* found that strong social support plays a protective role against depression. Regular interaction with friends and family members can act as a buffer against feelings of isolation and loneliness, common precursors to depression. Arrange to meet up with a friend for coffee or a walk, or set aside time for a regular catch-up call with a family member or join a coaching programme that offers group coaching calls. See chapter 17 on relationships.

Attitude of gratitude: Keeping a gratitude journal can also be a valuable tool. Research in the *Journal of Happiness Studies* showed that regularly jotting down things you're grateful for can lead to lower levels of depression and higher levels of well-being.

I have a range of gratitude journals for sale on my website and on Amazon if you want to take a look, but even just a plain notebook will do if you don't need prompts.

Mind the gap: Mindfulness and meditation can also play a significant role. Mindfulness-based cognitive therapy (MBCT) can reduce symptoms of depression by helping individuals become aware of their thoughts and feelings and making it easier to break the cycle of depression and relapse.

I've found in my coaching practice, that learning what elevates your moods, and what drains them, is super beneficial too. In addition, reflecting on which humans in your life uplift you, and which are Debbie

Downers that steal your dreams and pop your spirit, is of utmost importance. If we are the average of the five people we hang around with the most, choose them carefully.

One more piece of advice is to put yourself on top of your priority list and make sure that you are doing something for yourself each, and every, day. I call this 'feeding your fairy' (not a euphemism). It's a core principle that is so vital to a positive and buoyant mindset.

If your symptoms are severe and persistent, it's important to consult a healthcare provider for a tailored treatment plan, which may include medication or other therapies.

Depression during perimenopause is a multi-faceted issue, but it's crucial to know that it's manageable. From exercise and social support to dietary changes and mindfulness, there are various avenues you can explore to improve your mental well-being. Remember, you're not alone, and help is available.

Mood Swings

Mood swings during perimenopause can sometimes feel like you have multiple personalities and nearly all of them are royally pissed off! One moment, you're floating on cloud nine, thrilled about a recent achievement or a simple yet lovely interaction. But before you know it, you're plummeting into a pit of despair, irritated at the drop of a hat, or engulfed in an emotional fog that just won't lift. It's not just disorienting for you; it's also a challenge for those who share your living space, work environment, or even just a coffee catch-up. Your fluctuating moods may perplex and worry them, not to mention it puts a strain on your relationships.

Now, while mood swings might feel like rogue waves overturning your emotional boat, there's a reason behind this choppy sea. Research published in the *Journal of Clinical Endocrinology and Metabolism* has shown that hormone imbalances, particularly involving oestrogen, play a significant role in mood disorders. Given that perimenopause is a time of hormonal tumult, it stands to reason that your moods may be more unpredictable than a British summer.

It's not all doom and gloom, though. Understanding the underlying reasons can empower you to take effective measures.

Self-Help Strategies

Mood Journal: Keeping track of your emotions might sound tedious, but it can be incredibly enlightening. There are user-friendly apps that allow you to log your moods, note triggers, and even correlate your emotional fluctuations with your menstrual cycle. For those who prefer good old pen and paper, a notebook will do the trick. Make a point to jot down not just your moods, but also the events, interactions, and thoughts that seem to precede mood changes. This self-observation can offer you valuable insights into patterns and triggers, ultimately enabling you to prepare for or even sidestep certain mood swings.

Regular Exercise: We can't stress this enough. Exercise is like a Swiss Army knife for mental health. It can aid sleep, boost your energy levels, and significantly stabilise your moods. The Mayo Clinic, as well as numerous studies, suggest that just thirty minutes a day can bring about noticeable improvements in mental well-being. And don't worry, you don't have to suddenly become a gym rat; activities like swimming, cycling, or even a spirited dance session in your living room can make a world of difference.

Nutritional Choices: It might sound cliché and somewhat repetitive throughout this book, but you really are what you eat, especially when it comes to your emotional state. Omega-3 fatty acids, found in fish like salmon and mackerel, have shown promise in balancing mood, according to research published in the *Journal of Clinical Psychiatry*. Similarly, foods rich in vitamin B6 can help with serotonin production, offering another line of defence against mood swings.

Mindfulness and Relaxation Techniques: The benefits of mindfulness meditation in mood regulation have been well-documented. Setting aside even a few minutes a day to meditate can help you become aware of your thoughts and feelings and make it easier to control your mood swings.

Talk About It: Sometimes talking through your emotions can offer a different perspective. Choose a confidant from your inner circle who you know will offer empathy and under-standing. Sometimes, venting or merely articulating what you're going through can lighten your emotional load.

Taking proactive steps to understand and manage your mood swings can change them from being a tumultuous torrent to a navigable stream. Remember, perimenopause is just a phase, but how you handle it can set the tone for the years to come. Take charge now, and you'll not just weather the storm but perhaps even enjoy the rainbow that follows.

Insomnia

Insomnia during perimenopause can leave you absolutely knackered. It's a particularly sneaky one because it doesn't just affect your night; it bleeds into your day, affecting your mood, concentration, and overall mental health. The Sleep Foundation notes that a staggering 40% of perimenopausal women struggle with sleep disturbances. This statistic is not just a number; it's a loud wake-up call (ironically) about the seriousness of sleep issues during this phase.

Sleep disturbances aren't merely an inconvenience; they're a significant health concern. *The Lancet Psychiatry* has published a study suggesting a strong association between insomnia and a range of mental health problems like depression and anxiety. Moreover, it's a vicious cycle: the more stressed or anxious you are about not sleeping, the harder it becomes to actually fall asleep. Add to these hormonal fluctuations that are already playing havoc with your emotional state, and it's clear why insomnia is such a pressing issue during perimenopause.

Now, the question is, what to do about it? Life might be throwing you some curveballs, but that doesn't mean you can't hit back.

Self-Help Strategies

Create a Sleep Sanctuary: If your bedroom currently feels more like an extension of your living room or workspace, it's time to reclaim it as your sleep haven. Block out light with blackout curtains, or if that's not feasible, an eye mask can be a helpful alternative. Make sure the room is cool; the Sleep Council recommends a temperature range of 16-18 degrees Celsius for optimal sleep conditions. The objective here is to create a dark, quiet, and cool environment that signals to your body it's time to wind down.

Mind Your Tech: This is crucial – take all electronic devices out of your bedroom. The blue light emitted by phones, tablets, and laptops is proven to interfere with melatonin production, the hormone responsible for regulating sleep. So, the 'quick' email check or social media scroll before bed is, in reality, an invitation to insomnia. Consider replacing your electronic devices with a good, old-fashioned book or perhaps some soothing music to lull you to sleep.

Weighted Blankets and White Noise Machines: These might sound like wellness fads, but they've gained popularity for a reason. A study in the *Journal of Clinical Sleep Medicine* has shown that weighted blankets can improve sleep quality. Similarly, white noise machines can mask environmental sounds, helping your brain relax and make the shift into sleep mode.

Mindfulness and Relaxation Techniques: A systematic review published in the *Annals of the New York Academy of Sciences* revealed that mindfulness meditation could improve sleep quality. Just a few minutes of deep breathing, progressive muscle relaxation, or a quick mindfulness meditation session can prepare your body and mind for restful sleep.

Nutrition and Caffeine: Beware of food and drink that can sabotage your sleep. Caffeine stays in your system for up to six hours, so that afternoon coffee could be the culprit behind your sleeplessness. Opt for caffeine-free herbal teas like chamomile or valerian root in the evening.

Routine, Routine, Routine: It might sound dull, but having a regular sleep schedule – even on weekends – can significantly improve your sleep quality. Consistency helps regulate your body's internal clock and could help you fall asleep and wake up more easily.

Brain Dumping. If you find yourself tossing and turning at night, with a whirlwind of thoughts keeping you awake, you're not alone. Insomnia is a common companion during perimenopause, but one effective strategy for tackling it is a 'brain dump' before bedtime. Picture it as a decluttering exercise for your mind. Grab a notebook and jot down everything that's on your mind – worries, to-do lists, unresolved issues, random thoughts, you name it. By transferring these thoughts onto paper, you essentially offload them from your mind, giving yourself permission to mentally step away. Research published in the *Journal of Experimental Psychology* found that people who wrote down their to-dos before sleep fell asleep faster than those who didn't. So, as you navigate the sleep challenges of perimenopause, give your brain a good old-fashioned clear-out. It's like tidying up your mental living room before settling down for a peaceful night's sleep.

You might not solve your sleep issues overnight, but taking these steps will move you closer to regaining those precious hours of rest. A good night's sleep is not just a luxury; it's a necessity for your well-being, especially during this pivotal life stage.

Don't just count sheep; make your sleep count.

Panic Attacks

Panic attacks during perimenopause can feel like a horrible surprise. They can swoop in out of nowhere, sending you into a spiral of terrifying symptoms that often resemble more severe health issues. It's no wonder that panic attacks can send you into, well, a panic! According to NHS data, one in ten people experience occasional panic attacks, which makes it a not-so-uncommon issue, although it can feel intensely isolating when it happens to you.

A panic attack is not merely an emotional response but also a physiological one, involving a surge of adrenaline that puts your body in a hyper-vigilant state. This can lead to symptoms like rapid heart rate, shortness of breath, and even a sense of impending doom. It can be a frightening experience, and knowing that hormone fluctuations during perimenopause can exacerbate these symptoms doesn't make it any easier.

The good news is, while panic attacks are scary, they're usually not medically dangerous. A study published in the *British Journal of Psychiatry* confirms that cognitive behavioural therapy (CBT) is effective in treating panic disorders, but even before you consider something as structured as CBT, there are steps you can take right at the moment a panic attack strikes.

Self-Help Strategies

Breathing Techniques: The first line of defence during a panic attack is your breath. A technique often recommended by psychologists involves square breathing or the 4-4-4-4 rule. Inhale deeply through your nose for four counts, hold the breath for another four counts, exhale through your mouth for four counts, and then hold your breath again for four counts. This technique not only calms your nervous system but also distracts your mind from the panic symptoms. Repeating this cycle can help you regain emotional equilibrium.

Grounding Techniques: If you feel disconnected during a panic attack, grounding techniques can bring you back to the present moment. Engage your senses by identifying five things you can see, four things you can touch, three things you can hear, two things you can smell, and one thing you can taste. This sensory exercise can shift your focus from internal turmoil to external stimuli, providing an emotional 'anchor.'

Pause and Locate: Take a moment to locate yourself physically. Feel your feet on the ground or your hands touching a surface. This simple act can be surprisingly effective in detaching you from the emotional intensity of a panic attack. It's like telling your brain, "Look, we are here, we are grounded, we are safe."

Safe Space Imagery: Close your eyes and visualise a place that brings you peace. It could be a beach, a forest, or even a memorable room from your past. Engage all your senses in this visualisation. What do you see, hear, or smell? This form of mental escape can help in reducing the symptoms of a panic attack.

Call a Friend: Sometimes the quickest way to defuse a panic attack is to engage in a casual conversation with a friend or family member. The act of talking can be a wonderful distraction, plus it has the added benefit of human connection, reminding you that you're not alone.

Professional Help: While self-help techniques are valuable, recurrent panic attacks may require the expertise of an experienced coach or healthcare provider. You don't have to battle them on your own. I have an anxiety journal on my website with QR codes you can scan to go to the training video for each exercise.

Navigating panic attacks, particularly during perimenopause, is no small feat. But remember, these attacks are time-limited; they will pass. Each step you take to manage your symptoms is a step toward reclaiming your emotional wellbeing.

Irritability

Irritability during perimenopause is a common experience and can manifest as a low tolerance for things that you might usually brush off, causing you to react more strongly or emotionally than usual. The fluctuations in hormones like oestrogen and progesterone contribute to this heightened emotional state. If you find yourself snapping at loved ones or getting frustrated over little things, know that you're not alone.

Why do you feel irritable? Well, hormone imbalances can significantly affect neurotransmitters in your brain. This can lead to irritability or even mood swings. In some instances, poor sleep quality, also a hallmark of perimenopause, can contribute to a short temper. According to the National Sleep Foundation, lack of sleep can significantly worsen mood and contribute to a reduced threshold for stress.

Exercise can be an excellent tool in combating irritability. Harvard Health Publishing indicates that engaging in aerobic exercise for just twenty to thirty minutes a day can produce mood-improving endorphins, which are natural chemicals in the brain that act like painkillers and mood elevators. Not only does it give you a chance to clear your head, but it can also improve sleep quality, tackling two birds with one stone.

But exercise alone may not be sufficient. Identifying specific irritants or triggers in your environment can also be instrumental in managing irritability. You could find that certain foods or drinks, particularly those high in sugar or caffeine, may exacerbate your symptoms. Keeping a food diary could provide valuable insights into which substances make you feel more irritable. Track what you eat alongside your mood to see if you notice any patterns.

Another useful technique is to engage in mindfulness practices or meditation to bring your awareness back to the present. According to a 2010 meta-analytic review, mindfulness-based therapy can improve symptoms of anxiety, depression, and irritability. Mindfulness can help you become aware of your emotions and triggers, giving you an opportunity to choose how to react rather than responding impulsively.

And don't forget, while it might feel like you're on an emotional roller coaster, this phase is temporary. Engage in open conversations with your loved ones about what you're going through. The support and understanding of your close circle can be invaluable during this time, offering not just emotional comfort but also perspective when things feel overwhelming.

Self-Help Strategies

Exercise: Consider setting aside time for regular exercise; it could be something as simple as a twenty-minute walk around the neighbourhood or a home-based workout. Consistency is key.

Food and/or Diary: Use a food and mood diary to track possible irritants and think about incorporating mindfulness practices into your daily routine.

Mindfulness: Just ten minutes of mindfulness meditation can make a noticeable difference in your mood.

Support Circle: Lastly, keep your support circle informed and engaged; their understanding and support can provide you with an emotional cushion against irritability.

Stress

Stress is like the invisible backpack we all carry around, and unfortunately, during perimenopause, it often feels like someone's added a few more bricks to it. Suddenly, deciding what's for dinner can feel like you're defusing a bomb. You're not alone; stress is a common companion of perimenopause.

The Causes

You guessed it – hormones are at it again. Just like they did in our teen-age years, hormones during perimenopause seem determined to rock the emotional boat. The fluctuating levels of oestrogen and progester-one can directly affect the stress hormone, cortisol. No wonder your nerves might be more frayed than a well-worn dishcloth.

Stress is so ubiquitous that it's hard to pin down exact figures for how many perimenopausal women are affected. However, according to the Mental Health Foundation, 74% of UK adults have felt so stressed at some point over the last year they felt overwhelmed or unable to cope. The overlap with perimenopausal symptoms just adds an extra layer to the stress cake. And no, it's not a cake anyone wants a slice of.

Consult a Healthcare Provider if your stress levels are consistently off the charts. Chronic stress is linked to a variety of health issues, such as high blood pressure, diabetes, and mental health problems. A healthcare provider can guide you through medical solutions or even recommend a specialist, like a life coach or counsellor, for cognitive be-havioural therapy or other stress-reducing methods. Stress is some-thing I probably speak about in more client calls than not and it's some-thing that is very detrimental to so many women's lives.

Self-Help Strategies

Time Management: Techniques like the Pomodoro Technique can turn mountains into molehills by breaking tasks into manageable bites. Less daunting tasks = less stress.

Mindfulness: This is more than a buzzword; mindfulness can actually help rewire stress reactions in the brain. Meditation, even just five to ten minutes a day, can significantly lower stress levels.

Physical Activity: Physical exercise releases endorphins, aka the feel-good hormones. No need to become an Olympic athlete – simple exer-cises like walking can have substantial benefits.

Eat Right: Avoid caffeine and sugar, the impostors of energy. Instead, opt for a balanced diet rich in fruits, vegetables, and lean proteins to keep your blood sugar stable and your stress at bay.

Natural Remedies: Chamomile, lavender, and even CBD oil are claimed to have stress-reducing properties. Always consult with a healthcare provider before adding new supplements to your routine. Valerian root I have found personally really helps too.

Deep Breathing: It sounds too simple to be effective, but deep breathing exercises like the 4-7-8 method can be surprisingly effective in calming the nervous system. Or try the Cocoa Breaths exercise (video on my YouTube channel).

Set Boundaries: Whether it's saying no to extra responsibilities or taking time off social media, setting limits can help manage stress.

Connect: Don't underestimate the power of a good chinwag with a friend or loved one. Sometimes talking it out can be the best medicine.

It may seem like your stress, on a scale of 1 to 10, where 1 is a chilled bunny and 10 is rampant rage, has been dialled up to 11 during perimenopause, but remember, this isn't your first rodeo. You've managed stress before, and with some new strategies in your toolkit, you can manage it now.

Feeling Dead Inside
The feeling of being 'dead inside' or emotionally numb is a significant concern, particularly during perimenopause when you're already dealing with a host of physical and emotional changes. This numbing sensation can envelop you like a dense fog, making even the simple tasks seem meaningless and robbing you of the ability to feel joy, sadness, or any emotion in between.

One contributing factor is hormonal imbalances, common during peri-menopause. Hormones like serotonin, which are responsible for regulating mood, can fluctuate during this period. The imbalance can lead to feelings of emotional flatlining.

Another reason could be burnout. Many women in their 40s and 50s are juggling multiple responsibilities – career, family, possibly caregiving for elderly parents. The sustained stress can make you emotionally and mentally exhausted, leading to this disconcerting numbness.

Then there's the existential aspect. With children possibly moving out and the prospect of retirement on the horizon, you might be facing an identity crisis. Who are you when you're not fulfilling your usual roles? This questioning can plunge you into emotional apathy as a self-protective mechanism.

It's also worth noting that feeling emotionally numb can be a symptom of more serious mental health conditions, like depression or anxiety disorders. In a 2018 study published in the journal *Menopause*, about 16.6% of perimenopausal women met the criteria for at least one depressive disorder.

Please consult a medical specialist or healthcare provider if you are worried about your symptoms.

Self-Help Strategies
Firstly, it's vital to recognise that this emotional numbness is not an end but a symptom, signalling a need for self-care and perhaps professional help.

Let's Build on the Idea of Re-engagement: |My philosophy here is simple but profound: "Your motion creates your emotion." Start with activities that required minimal effort but gave you a sense of accomplishment or happiness in the past. It could be something as straightforward as walking in the park, doodling, cooking a meal, or even arranging a bouquet of flowers. According to my own research, engaging in creative activities leads to increased well-being and a more positive state of mind.

Break it Down: Another step is to break down your daily tasks into smaller, manageable parts. I have found that breaking tasks down increases the likelihood of engaging in activities and reduces feelings of overwhelm, thereby helping to improve emotional regulation.

Friends and Family: Don't underestimate the power of social support. Sometimes, the way out of your own head is through meaningful connections. Research published in the *Journal of Psychosomatic Research* found a strong association between social support and emotional well-being. Even if you're not up for socialising, a simple phone call with a close friend or family member can sometimes lift the fog, even just a bit.

Breathe...: Breathing exercises can also be helpful. Slow breathwork can reduce symptoms of psychological distress, including feelings of emotional numbness.

Remember, there's no 'one size fits all,' so it's okay if some steps work better for you than others. The crucial part is to take action, no matter how small. Your emotional health is worth investing in, especially during a transitional phase like perimenopause. You're not alone, and it's never too late to seek help and re-engage with your life emotionally.

Emotional Vulnerability

Emotional vulnerability during perimenopause can feel like you're walking on a tightrope without a safety net. One minute you're perfectly fine, and the next, you're welling up over a sentimental advert. It's like your emotional filters have gone on the fritz, making you more susceptible to feeling raw or exposed. Again, don't give yourself a hard time over it; this emotional sensitivity is partly due to hormone shifts affecting neurotransmitters that regulate mood and emotional response.

Understanding your emotional vulnerability is the first step in navigating it. We often perceive vulnerability as a weakness when, in reality, it's a natural human experience that allows for deeper connections with others and ourselves. It's the cornerstone of empathy, compassion, and even love. So, if you find yourself tearing up more often or feeling emotionally 'naked,' it's okay. You're not falling apart; you're just tuning into a richer emotional landscape, one that can be incredibly rewarding if navigated wisely.

Self-Help Strategies

Labels: Start by practising emotional labelling whenever you feel particularly vulnerable. Take a deep breath and identify what you're feeling. Write it down if it helps. Then, try sharing these feelings with someone you're close to, whether it's a friend, a family member, or even a healthcare professional. It's like emotional weightlifting – the more you do it, the stronger your emotional resilience will become. After all, vulnerability isn't about weakness; it's about the courage to experience life fully, highs and lows included.

Talk About It: Keeping your emotions bottled up isn't healthy Another method is to confide in someone you trust. There's a transformative power in sharing your emotions openly, and it can be a therapeutic exercise in itself. Your perimenopausal journey might be a personal one, but that doesn't mean you have to go through it alone. Reach out and be honest about your feelings. You'll be surprised how much lighter you feel by simply voicing what's going on inside you.

Cognitive Behavioural Therapy (CBT) Techniques: These tools can help you reframe negative thought patterns. You don't necessarily need to see a therapist to start practicing CBT techniques; there are many self-help books and online resources available including the journal that goes along with this book.

Emotion Regulation Skills: Techniques like mindfulness and deep-breathing exercises can help you manage intense emotions. The more you practice, the easier it will become to keep your cool.

Lifestyle Influences: Exercise is a powerful tool for managing mood swings and emotional vulnerability. Even a simple thirty-minute walk each day can work wonders.

Your diet can directly affect your mood. Make sure to eat balanced meals rich in protein, fibre, and healthy fats. Avoid excess sugar and caffeine, which can exacerbate mood swings. Lack of sleep can also worsen emotional vulnerability. Aim for seven to eight hours of quality sleep each night.

Support Groups: Sometimes speaking to others who are going through the same thing can provide emotional relief and useful coping mechanisms. Feel free to add yourself to my free support group on Facebook called "Perimenopause with Kate Grosvenor." It's fabulous for asking questions, supporting others, reading other people's stories and knowing that you are truly not alone.

CHAPTER 29

Healing Level 4

Mindset Issues

A long with the discussion on mental health, comes a chapter on mindset issues too – a space that's as important to navigate as the hot flushes and irregular periods. We'll explore a range of mindset issues many women experience, from low self-esteem and sh*t FM (negative self-talk) to bouts of imposter syndrome a distinct lack of motivation.

You're not alone if you've felt like a different version of yourself or wondered why your get-up-and-go seems to have buggered-off-and-gone. Thankfully, awareness is the first step toward positive change, and there are effective strategies to help you manage your mindset during this transitional time. So, let's embark on this enlightening journey together, filled with helpful insights, practical tips, and the encouraging reminder that you can tackle these challenges with grace and resilience. The road of perimenopause may be winding, but it also leads to new vistas of self-discovery and empowerment.

Low Self-Esteem

Low self-esteem during perimenopause is an all-too-common issue that countless women grapple with, yet it's seldom discussed openly. As your body goes through significant changes, your self-image may be shaken, and it can feel like you've lost a part of your identity. This phase of life is accompanied by physical symptoms like weight gain, hot flashes, and changes in skin texture, all of which can take a toll on how you feel about yourself. While it's natural to associate a large part of your identity with your physical self, these changes can make you question your worth or desirability.

Another contributing factor to low self-esteem during this period is societal expectations. We live in a culture that often prizes youth and overlooks the beauty and wisdom that come with age. The media's relentless focus on youthfulness can make you feel 'past your prime,' even though age should be celebrated as an emblem of experience and wisdom.

Work and career transitions can further fuel low self-esteem. Many women in their 40s and 50s are at the peak of their career, but the pressure to stay at the top of your game while also dealing with perimenopausal symptoms can be daunting. You might be dealing with younger colleagues climbing the corporate ladder quickly, which can make you feel like you're being left behind.

Let's not forget the emotional toll. Perimenopause often coincides with significant life events like children leaving home for college or parents requiring more care. These changes can leave you feeling emotionally empty and question your role and worth, contributing to a decline in self-esteem.

Self-Help Strategies
One crucial step in rebuilding your self-esteem is to practise self-compassion. Treat yourself with the same kindness and understanding as you would a good friend. A study published in the journal *Mindfulness and Self-Compassion* found that self-compassion exercises could lead to an immediate improvement in mood and self-esteem.

Exercise is another powerful tool for improving self-esteem. Physical activity releases endorphins, often referred to as 'feel-good hormones.' Research in the *Journal of Sports Sciences* has shown that regular physical exercise can significantly improve self-esteem and mental well-being. So, whether it's yoga, walking, or dancing in your living room, make time for activities that make you feel alive.

Also, consider joining or creating a support group. Sometimes, just knowing that you're not alone in your experiences can be incredibly empowering. Social support can significantly improve self-esteem and mental well-being.

Finally, don't shy away from seeking professional guidance. Life coaches and therapists can provide you with coping mechanisms tailored specifically for you. Cognitive behavioural therapy, for example, is a proven method for improving self-esteem by challenging and changing your destructive thoughts and behaviours.

Low self-esteem during perimenopause is a complex issue, but remember, it's just a chapter, not your whole story. With actionable steps and a compassionate approach, you can rewrite this chapter into one of empowerment and self-love.

Negative Self-Talk

Let's delve into the topic of "Sh*t FM" (the term I use to accurately describe the radio-like station in your mind that plays sh*t and negative self-talk to you all day). During perimenopause, an age and stage where it seems your internal radio station is on a loop of unhelpful tracks, the volume can seem particularly loud.

Negative self-talk can feel like an endless playlist of criticisms and doubts, and during perimenopause, it seems like the volume knob is broken – stuck on loud. It's a turbulent time when your body is undergoing hormonal changes, and the side effects aren't just physical; they're mental and emotional too. The fluctuation in hormones can lead to mood swings, irritability, and even depression, which can all serve as background music to this damaging inner dialogue.

So, why does the radio station in your head lean toward the negative? There's actually a scientific term for this: 'negativity bias'. Negative events have a greater impact on our psychological state than neutral or positive events. This bias might have served us well in evolutionary terms, making us alert to potential dangers, but in modern-day life, it often just results in a heavy rotation of self-criticism and pessimism.

Self-Help Strategies

Mindfulness: It's time to turn down "Sh*t FM" and tune into a more empowering station. One way to do this is through mindfulness meditation. Mindfulness can significantly reduce negative self-talk and improve overall emotional well-being. Another method is to actively challenge your inner critic. Every time you catch yourself engaging in negative self-talk, counter it with a positive or more realistic statement. For example, change "I'll never get this right" to "I can learn and improve with practice".

Positive Affirmations: There's also something incredibly powerful about actually writing down the positive affirmations. Writing down positive experiences or affirmations can enhance your positive outlook and even contribute to better mental health. So, start journaling the 'hits' instead of the 'misses' to help reprogram your internal radio station.

And sometimes, it can be beneficial to talk it out with someone you trust or get professional help with a life coach. Social support could play a significant role in diminishing negative self-talk. When you externalise what's playing on your internal radio, often you realise that the playlist isn't rooted in reality.

So, there you have it. Turning down "Sh*t FM" and tuning into a channel that uplifts you is not an overnight task, but it is certainly doable.

With some conscious effort and strategic steps, you can change the station and turn the volume down on the negativity, leading to a more harmonious life soundtrack.

Lack of Motivation

I call this the 'perimenopausal treacle walk,' a phase where you feel like you're wading through a thick, sticky mess both mentally and physically. Let's get something straight: this is not a character flaw, a lack of discipline, or a sign that you're 'letting yourself go.' This is a common experience that many women go through, and it's largely due to fluctuating hormones affecting everything from your mood to your energy levels.

Let's start with the science of it. Hormonal fluctuations during perimenopause can significantly impact neurotransmitters like serotonin, which plays a crucial role in regulating mood and motivation. Lower levels of serotonin can lead to feelings of sadness and reduced drive. It's like your internal pep squad has gone on a holiday, leaving you to navigate this phase on your own. But before you lose hope, remember that motivation ebbs and flows even under regular circumstances. During perimenopause, this just gets amplified.

The feeling of being overwhelmed is often what holds us back. The trick to overcoming this is to break everything down into smaller, more digestible tasks. For instance, instead of setting an ambitious goal like "I'll organise the entire house today," start with one drawer or one room. The scale may be smaller, but the sense of accomplishment will be just as fulfilling.

And yes, celebrate those small victories – because they matter. Acknowledging small wins can significantly boost your sense of competence, and by extension, your motivation. Even science backs the power of a mini celebration. So, if you've managed to clear out your email inbox, don't just shrug it off. Take a moment to bask in that achievement.

The same goes for going for a brisk walk or finishing a chapter of that book you've been meaning to read.

Self-Help Strategies
How Do You Eat an Elephant?: The answer is one bite at a time. Start by making a list of tasks you need to accomplish, and then break each of them down into smaller, more manageable actions.

Happy Dance: Every time you tick off a task, take a moment to celebrate, however you see fit – a happy dance, a cup of your favourite tea, or simply a few deep, satisfying breaths to acknowledge your achievement. These moments of recognition are not just fluff; they're scientifically proven motivational boosters.

So next time you find yourself knee-deep in metaphorical treacle, remember that every small step you take is a victory in reigniting your motivation. You're not stuck; you're just pacing yourself, gathering momentum for the next phase of your journey.**Fear of Change**
Fear of change can become especially pronounced during perimenopause. It's a time when you're already dealing with various physiological shifts, and the idea of additional change can feel overwhelming. However, it's important to remember that change isn't always your enemy; sometimes, it's an opportunity for growth and newfound freedom.

Self Help Strategies
Make Change Your Friend: To face this fear head-on, familiarise yourself with change. To help you navigate this fear, try to introduce minor changes into your daily routine.

Start small: Choose activities like rearranging your furniture, taking a different route to the supermarket, or trying a new recipe. So, consider starting with simple things, like taking a different route to the supermarket or trying a new recipe. These small changes can act as stepping stones, helping you build resilience and become more comfortable with larger life transitions.

A study in the *Journal of Experimental Social Psychology* found that people who embraced new experiences, even minor ones, showed higher overall well-being.

Procrastination

Procrastination is frequently misunderstood as mere laziness or poor time management, but it's often far more complex than that. Particularly during perimenopause, when hormone imbalances can send your stress levels skyrocketing, procrastination might be your brain's way of saying, "Hold on, this is too much for me right now".

In psychological terms, procrastination can be seen as a coping mechanism for stress and emotional overwhelm. When faced with a task that triggers anxiety or self-doubt, your brain might opt for the 'flight' in the 'fight or flight' response, steering you away from the source of stress. So, instead of writing that report, you might find yourself mindlessly scrolling through social media or organising your spice rack – tasks that are inconsequential in comparison but provide a temporary emotional refuge.

Self Help Strategies

Time-Boxing: One effective way to manage procrastination is by 'time-boxing,' where you allocate specific time slots to specific tasks. This gives you the structure and limits the mental load, making the task less overwhelming. Time management strategies like these can significantly reduce procrastination and related stress.

Journals Help: *The UncompliKated to Perimenopause Journal* that is a natural companion to this book can help you with task and to help you keep on track.

Do the Worst First: Another method to consider is the 'Worst-First' approach. Tackle the most daunting task first thing in the morning when your willpower is at its peak. Willpower operates like a muscle and is strongest when you have not exhausted it on other tasks.

The Two-Minute Rule: The 'two-minute rule' can be another game-changer here. If something takes less than two minutes, do it immediately. This is backed by the principle that the action of starting can often be harder than the task itself. Once you start, you're more likely to continue. Research from the University of Sheffield found that people are more likely to engage in a task once they've initiated it, even if it was reluctantly started.

The Pareto Principle: Another helpful technique is the 'Pareto Principle,' suggesting that 80% of outcomes result from 20% of all causes for any given event. In essence, focus on tasks that will produce significant results and deprioritise less impactful ones.

Understanding procrastination as more than just 'laziness' can also be emotionally liberating. Knowing that procrastination is often your mind's way of handling stress can make you more compassionate towards yourself, and that self-compassion can be the first step in breaking the cycle.

Imposter Syndrome

Imposter Syndrome isn't just a fleeting feeling of self-doubt; it's a pervasive belief that you're a fraud, undeserving of your success and accomplishments. This internalised fear can have a crippling impact on your work, relationships, and self-esteem. While Imposter Syndrome is a universal phenomenon, research indicates it disproportionately affects women. The hormonal fluctuations and emotional volatility often experienced during perimenopause can add another layer of complexity, making you even more susceptible to these intrusive thoughts.

Now, why does Imposter Syndrome seem to ramp up during perimenopause? One reason might be the social and cultural expectations placed on women in this age group. You're often expected to 'have it all together' by now, which only amplifies the pressure and fuels the fear of being exposed as a fraud. In a study published in the *International*

Journal of Behavioural Science, nearly 70% of participants reported experiencing feelings related to Imposter Syndrome, indicating how prevalent this issue is, especially among high achievers.

Self-Help Strategies

Reframing: One effective strategy to combat Imposter Syndrome is through 'reframing,' a cognitive behavioural technique. Instead of viewing your role or task as something you could potentially fail at, see it as a learning opportunity. When you switch the focus from performance to learning, the fear of failure becomes less intimidating.

Check Your Underlying Beliefs: Another valuable method is to identify and to question the underlying beliefs that fuel your Imposter Syndrome. Are you setting unrealistically high standards for yourself? Are you attributing your success to external factors like luck or timing, instead of acknowledging your skills and efforts? A study in the *Journal of Rational-Emotive & Cognitive-behaviour Therapy* found that challenging these core beliefs could reduce symptoms of Imposter Syndrome.

Find a Mentor: Don't underestimate the power of mentorship either. Connecting with someone who has walked the path before you can provide valuable perspectives that can debunk some of the myths feeding your Imposter Syndrome. A study from the *Journal of Vocational Behaviour* found that mentorship significantly reduced career-related anxiety and bolstered self-esteem.

Achievement Journal: And here's a simple yet powerful tip: keep an 'achievement journal.' Whenever you hit a milestone, however minor, jot it down. According to a study published in the *Journal of Behavioural Science*, regularly documenting your achievements can boost your confidence and serve as a tangible counter-narrative to your imposter thoughts. *The UncompliKated Guide to Perimenopause Journal* is great for recording 'wins' – no matter how small.

Keeping a dedicated 'wins' journal to record everything you accomplish, no matter how trivial will not only serve as a personal reminder of your skills and successes, but it will also provide a valuable resource for future job applications or performance reviews.

Conquering Imposter Syndrome is rarely a quick fix but consider it a work in progress. Each step you take is a step away from self-doubt and a step closer to self-assurance. During perimenopause, you've got enough on your plate, so isn't it time you started serving yourself a slice of self-compassion and recognition? You've earned it.

Feeling Stuck

Feeling stuck can be incredibly challenging, particularly during perimenopause when your body is already going through so many changes. The sensation of being unable to move forward in aspects of your life – whether career, personal development, or relationships – can take a toll on your mental well-being. You're not alone in this. According to a study published in the *Journal of Epidemiology and Community Health*, women in their 40s and 50s are more likely than younger women to experience feelings of life dissatisfaction and being 'stuck.'

Now, why do you feel stuck? While hormone imbalances during perimenopause can affect mood, your feelings might also be influenced by external factors such as career plateaus, relationship issues, or the challenges of parenting, often with teenagers or adult children. Moreover, societal expectations can put pressure on women in this age group, making you feel that you should have 'achieved' certain things by now. The weight of these expectations combined with biological changes can exacerbate this feeling of stagnation.

Self Help Strategies

Shake it Off: Exercise can offer some relief by helping to release endorphins and giving you a sense of accomplishment, however small.

Quick Wins: What may be even more beneficial are 'quick wins,' those small, manageable tasks or achievements that might seem insignificant in the grand scheme of things but can make a world of difference to your mindset.

Quick wins can boost morale and increase your confidence, proving that you're capable of progress, even if it's just in small steps. These quick wins could be as simple as sorting out a cluttered drawer, finishing a book, or even learning a new recipe. The idea is to set achievable goals that lead to immediate rewards, creating a positive feedback loop that motivates you to tackle bigger challenges over time.

Mindfulness: Mindfulness and gratitude practices can also be potent in battling feelings of being stuck. Rather than focusing on what's not moving, bring your attention to what you have achieved and what's going well in your life. Practicing gratitude can increase well-being and life satisfaction and is something I talk about a lot with my clients.

CBT: If you find that you're stuck in negative thought patterns, cognitive behavioural therapy (CBT) techniques could be beneficial. A study in the *British Journal of Psychiatry* supports the effectiveness of CBT for improving mood and emotional well-being, teaching you to replace irrational thoughts with more balanced and constructive ones.

Begin by identifying a few quick wins — tasks you can complete in a day or less that will bring you some level of satisfaction. Aim to accomplish at least one or two a week and celebrate these small victories. Engage in mindfulness or gratitude exercises daily to shift your focus from what's not working to what is. And, if you find that you're overwhelmed by negative thoughts, consider CBT techniques or online courses designed to challenge and alter unproductive thought patterns. The key is to take small, proactive steps to change your mental landscape, laying the groundwork for bigger shifts in your life.

Emotional Eating

Emotional eating during perimenopause can feel like a double whammy. Your hormones are already playing a symphony of mood swings, and now they're also conducting your eating habits. It's a challenge that many women in their 40s and beyond face. According to a study published in the journal *Menopause*, nearly 40% of perimenopausal women have increased eating behaviours, including emotional eating. It's not just about hunger; emotional eating often serves as a coping mechanism for stress, sadness, or even boredom, and the hormonal imbalances associated with perimenopause can exacerbate this tendency.

Why does this happen? Emotional eating can be attributed to various factors, including fluctuating serotonin levels, which can influence your mood and appetite. When you're emotionally charged, the brain often craves 'comfort foods' rich in sugar, fat, and carbohydrates to temporarily elevate serotonin levels, providing a fleeting sense of relief. But these effects are short-lived and often followed by feelings of guilt or more emotional turbulence, creating a vicious cycle.

Another contributing factor can be societal expectations. Women are often conditioned to suppress emotional outbursts, so instead of venting, you might find solace in food. The taboos surrounding discussions about perimenopause may also mean you turn to food instead of seeking emotional support. It's as if you're navigating a minefield blindfolded, and the only guide you have is a tub of ice cream.

Self-Help Strategies

The good news is there are ways to manage emotional eating effectively.

Mindfulness Techniques: These can be a game-changer in helping you understand the emotions that trigger binge eating. Mindfulness-based interventions can significantly reduce emotional eating by training you to be more aware of what you're feeling when you reach for that extra cookie. Is it hunger, or is it sadness, stress, or loneliness? Being able to distinguish between emotional and physical hunger is the first step towards making healthier choices.

Meal Planning: It's not just mindfulness that can help; structured meal planning can also break the cycle. Plan balanced meals and snacks ahead of time to avoid last-minute, emotion-driven eating decisions. Knowing what and when you'll eat next can help you regain a sense of control.

Create a Master Meal Plan: List down balanced meals and snacks and stick to this plan as much as possible. This is especially helpful if you have children at home. Brainstorm a list of meals everyone agrees on and then simply rotate as you like. It saves that constant question "what are you in the mood for?"

Support: Moreover, don't underestimate the power of a strong support network. Social support can positively influence weight-loss outcomes. It's much easier to turn away from emotional eating when you have friends or family to talk through your worries and frustrations.

Comparititis

Ah, the infamous 'Comparison Trap,' or as I term it, 'comparititis' – the disease of the soul you get from comparing yourself to other women. This condition seems to spike around perimenopause, a time when life is already throwing enough curveballs. Comparing yourself to others is an age-old habit, but the advent of social media has turned it into a full-blown epidemic. Scroll through your Instagram feed, and suddenly, everyone's life looks perfect, their relationships sublime, and don't even get me started on the age-defying selfies.

And guess what? Comparititis doesn't just affect your mental state; it can spill over into your physical health as well. A 2017 study published in the *Psychological Bulletin* found that frequent social comparison is associated with negative health outcomes, including increased stress, a higher risk of depression, and even compromised immune function. The kicker? The study also indicated that the effects were more pronounced in women compared to men.

How does this happen? Our brains are hardwired to create benchmarks. Comparisons can provide a context that might be beneficial in some scenarios – like in competitive sports or academics. But apply that to personal life and achievements, and it becomes a slippery slope. During perimenopause, this becomes even more pronounced because you're already grappling with physical changes, making you more susceptible to this comparison game. Your internal critic comes out to play, overshadowing your achievements and positive qualities. Before you know it, you're in a vortex of self-doubt, insecurity, and unhappiness.

The most insidious part about social media is that it's all an illusion, yet it feels so real. Rarely do people post about their struggles, their less-than-picture-perfect relationships, or the crow's feet they've been agonising over. All you see is a meticulously curated highlight reel that exacerbates your comparititis symptoms.

Self-Help Strategies
Reality: The first step towards healing is recognising the trap for what it is – a distorted view of reality.

Digital Detox: Take a digital detox or at least limit your exposure to platforms that fuel this incessant need for comparison. According to a 2019 study published in *JAMA Paediatrics*, high social media usage correlates directly with heightened internalising behaviours – another term for turning negative emotions inward, which can lead to mental health problems. Allocate specific times of the day for social media if going cold turkey seems daunting.

Feed Your Soul: Instead of scrolling aimlessly, engage in activities that bring joy and a sense of competence. Whether it's picking up a hobby, focusing on a project, or spending quality time with loved ones, these activities will not only divert your attention but also contribute to building a more robust self-image. It's all about creating a sense of self-worth that isn't contingent on external validation. By refocusing your energies, you begin to construct an internal fortress that is impervious to the trappings of external comparison. After all, the only person you should be in competition with is yourself, aiming for a happier, healthier version of who you are today.

CHAPTER 30

Recommended Supplements for Perimenopause

N avigating the maze of perimenopause can feel like a game of 3D chess – with your hormones making the moves! While the experience of perimenopause is as unique as you are, many women find that incorporating supplements into their wellness routine offers a valuable helping hand. As we journey through this chapter, we'll delve into the world of recommended supplements that could serve as your trusty sidekicks in this phase of life. From the popular heroes like black cohosh and evening primrose oil to lesser-known wonders like maca root, we'll break down what each supplement can do, how it interacts with your body, and what to keep an eye out for in terms of side effects.

But before we dive in, a little caveat: supplements are not a one-size-fits-all solution, and what works wonders for your best friend may not have the same magical effect on you. Always consult with a healthcare provider for personalised advice, especially if you're already on medication or have existing health conditions. Ready? Let's arm you with some knowledge so you can take on perimenopause like the empowered woman you are!

Ashwagandha:

Benefit: Helps to reduce stress and anxiety, which are common symptoms during perimenopause.

Recommended daily amount: 300-500 mg (standardised extract) but can vary based on the product and individual needs.

Note: Consult with a healthcare provider before combining with other supplements to avoid potential interactions.

Black Cohosh:

Benefit: Used traditionally to help with hot flashes and mood swings.

Recommended daily amount: 40-80 mg of a standardised extract, usually advised to be taken under medical supervision.

Note: Should not be taken with other liver-affecting substances without medical consultation due to potential liver toxicity.

Boron:

Benefit: Aids bone health, which can be compromised during perimenopause.

Recommended daily amount: 3-20 mg, depending upon dietary intake and individual needs.

Note: High doses can interfere with magnesium absorption; be cautious when taking alongside magnesium supplements.

Calcium:

Benefit: Essential for maintaining bone health during perimenopause.

Recommended daily amount: 1000-1300 mg, depending upon age and dietary intake.

Note: Best absorbed when taken with vitamin D; avoid taking with iron supplements as they can interfere with each other's absorption.

Chaste Tree (Vitex):

Benefit: May help in regulating menstrual cycles and alleviating mood swings.

Recommended daily amount: 20-40 mg of a standardised extract, under medical supervision.

Note: Should not be taken with hormonal contraceptives or hormone replacement therapy.

Dong Quai:

Benefit: Traditionally used to manage menstrual irregularities and symptoms of perimenopause.

Recommended daily amount: 500-2000 mg, although it is essential to follow the guidance of a healthcare provider.

Note: May increase sensitivity to sunlight and should not be combined with blood-thinning medications.

Evening Primrose Oil:

Benefit: Can potentially help with mood swings and hot flashes. Also known for alleviating symptoms like breast pain and promoting skin health.

Recommended daily amount: 500-1000 mg, though the dosage may vary.

Note: May interact with anticoagulant medications; consult with a healthcare provider if you are taking blood thinners.

Folic Acid:

Benefit: Supports overall health and may help prevent heart disease.

Recommended daily amount: 400-800 mcg, based on individual needs and dietary intake.

Note: Usually safe to take with other supplements but consult with a healthcare provider if you are taking medications for epilepsy or other neurological conditions.

Iron:

Benefit: Essential for preventing anaemia, especially in women experiencing heavy menstrual bleeding.

Recommended daily amount: 18 mg, though it may vary based on dietary iron intake and individual needs.

Note: Avoid taking with calcium supplements as they can interfere with each other's absorption.

Magnesium:

Benefit: Aids bone health and can help manage mood swings and sleep disturbances.

Recommended daily amount: 320 mg for women aged 31 and older.

Note: Can interact with certain medications including antibiotics and osteoporosis medications; consult a healthcare provider for guidance.

Maca Root:

Benefit: Enhances energy, stamina, and potentially reduces perimenopausal symptoms like hot flashes and disrupted sleep patterns.

Recommended daily amount: 1.5-3 grams of maca root powder is recommended but can vary based on individual needs and product specifications.

Note: If you are taking hormone-altering medications or supplements, consult with a healthcare provider before adding Maca to your regimen.

Milk Thistle

Benefit: Known for its liver-protective properties, it can aid in detoxifying the liver and may help to manage symptoms of hormonal imbalance experienced during perimenopause.

Recommended daily amount: 140-200 mg of silymarin (the active component in milk thistle) daily but consult with a healthcare provider for personalised guidance.

Note: May interact with medications metabolised by the liver; consult with a healthcare provider if you are taking medications, including blood thinners.

Omega-3 Fatty Acids:

Benefit: Helps in reducing inflammation and may aid in decreasing the risk of heart disease.

Recommended daily amount: 250-500 mg of combined EPA and DHA but can vary based on dietary intake and individual needs.

Note: May have blood-thinning effects; consult with a healthcare provider if you are taking blood thinners.

Probiotics:

Benefit: Can support gut health and the immune system.

Recommended daily amount: Varies widely, commonly ranging from 1 to 10 billion CFUs daily.

Note: Generally safe to take with other supplements but consult with a healthcare provider if you have a compromised immune system.

Starflower (Borage) Oil:

Benefit: Rich source of gamma-linolenic acid (GLA), potentially reducing symptoms like mood swings and irritability during perimenopause.

Recommended daily amount: Around 220-240 mg of GLA, generally considered safe and effective.

Note: May interact with anticoagulant medications; consult with a healthcare provider if you are taking blood thinners.

Vitamin B6:

Benefit: Can help in alleviating symptoms like irritability and depression associated with perimenopause.

Recommended daily amount: 1.3-1.7 mg, though it may vary based on age and individual needs.

Note: High doses can cause nerve damage; avoid taking with other supplements containing vitamin B6.

Vitamin B12:

Benefit: Important for maintaining energy levels and preventing anaemia.

Recommended daily amount: 2.4 mcg but can vary based on diet and individual needs.

Note: Generally safe to take with other supplements but consult with a healthcare provider if you have pernicious anaemia or other B12 absorption issues.

Vitamin C:

Benefit: Supports the immune system and is essential for collagen synthesis.

Recommended daily amount: 75 mg but can be higher based on individual needs and dietary intake.

Note: Can increase absorption of iron; avoid high doses as it may cause gastro-intestinal issues.

Vitamin D:

Benefit: Aids in calcium absorption and supports bone health.

Recommended daily amount: 600-800 IU but may be higher based on geographic location and individual needs.

Note: Best taken with calcium; consult with a healthcare provider if you are taking other supplements containing vitamin D.

Vitamin E:

Benefit: Can potentially help with vaginal dryness and hot flashes.

Recommended daily amount: 15 mg, but the dosage can vary based on individual needs and dietary intake.

Note: May interact with blood-thinning medications; consult with a healthcare provider if combining with other supplements.

Vitamin K:

Benefit: Works with Vitamin D and calcium to maintain bone health.

Recommended daily amount: 90 mcg, though it may vary based on diet and individual needs.

Note: Can interfere with blood-thinning medications; consult with a healthcare provider if you are on blood thinners.

Please consult with a healthcare provider to personalise a regimen that works best for you, especially considering potential interactions between supplements and any medications you may be taking.

** Disclaimer: The supplements discussed in this chapter are suggestions that some women have found helpful during the perimenopause stage. However, it is crucial to understand that I am not a healthcare provider, and the information provided should not be considered as medical advice.

Before adding and new supplements to your routine, it is imperative that you consult with a qualified healthcare professional for a personalised evaluation and recommendations. Your individual health needs, existing medical conditions, and current medications could interact with these supplements, making it essential to seek professional advice. Therefore, I cannot assume any responsibility for any outcomes related to the use of supplements mentioned. Always prioritise a consultation with a healthcare provider for the most accurate and personalised health advice and read the bottle before use for correct daily dose.

CHAPTER 31

The Journey Ahead

Let's Walk it Together

Hi, my lovely,

If you've made it as far as this chapter, then give yourself a massive pat on the back. You've navigated through the complex world of perimenopause and now you're on the other side of understanding, armed with insights, tips, and some good old wisdom. You know what they say: knowledge is power, but understanding is even better. Now that you're 'in the know,' it's time to use that newfound wisdom to better your life, and potentially even the lives of others. Let's not go it alone, shall we?

Further Resources, Just a Click Away!
I don't know about you, but I love a 'one-stop-shop' for resources. If you're keen to continue your journey of self-improvement and empowerment, I have a few things that you might be interested in:

One-to-One Coaching: Sometimes the best discoveries come through conversations. If you're looking to dig deeper, to have an accountability partner, or simply to chat about how to manage your next steps, my one-to-one coaching sessions could be just the ticket. It's like a tête-à-tête with a good friend, experienced coach, and a fellow perimenopausal woman who also knows more than a thing or two about your journey!

Group Coaching Programmes: Ah, the power of community! Imagine a place where women come together to share, to uplift, and to guide each other through the maze of perimenopause. Well, my group coaching programmes are that dream turned reality. Together, we're stronger.

My Other Books: If you've enjoyed *The UncompliKated Guide to Perimenopause*, you might like to explore some of my other publications. There is a journal, workbook and diary specifically designed to complement this book, giving you a more hands-on approach to tracking your progress and understanding your body. Jotting down your thoughts and observations can be surprisingly therapeutic. I also have anxiety journals, planners, notebooks and much more. These are all available on my website www.kategrosvenorbooks.com.

Facebook Support Group: I have a lovely group of like-minded women on Facebook – all of whom are going through this journey. The group is a place to ask questions, get (and give) support, and to know you are not on your own. Please note that I ask for your email address when you enter the group – you can choose to provide it or not – so that I can keep you up to date with any new resources or information, and to give you an idea of the programmes, workshops, and challenges that I run that would help you on your journey. You can just search for "Perimenopause with Kate Grosvenor" on Facebook and request to join the group.

Take the Next Step

Whether it's reaching out for coaching, diving into another book, or starting a journaling habit, taking that next step is crucial. If you're interested in any of the above, don't hesitate to visit my website or drop me an email.

To contact me:

- **Coaching Website**: www.kategrosvenor.com

- **Email**: kate@kategrosvenor.com

- **Discovery Call:** https://KateGrosvenorSchedule.as.me/DiscoveryCall

If you would like to join my **reading club** (Kate Grosvenor Reading Club) – where you get advanced sneak peaks of new publications, free book offers, and more you can go to www.kategrosvenorreadingclub.com . It's really worth signing up if you like books and journals on personal development, psychology/mindset, motivation, and more.

I want to leave you with a thought. Author Mary Anne Radmacher once said,

"Courage doesn't always roar.
Sometimes courage it's the quiet voice at the end of the day saying,
'I will try again tomorrow.'"

You don't have to conquer the world today or solve every issue in one go. Take small steps, but take them with courage. You're not alone on this journey; we're all walking this road together, one step at a time.

You're more resilient than you think, more capable than you know, and more amazing than you give yourself credit for. If you've picked up this book, you've already taken a step towards a better, more informed life. Now, keep walking. After all, the road ahead looks a lot better when you're striding down it with confidence and a few good friends, doesn't it?

Together we rise.

Buckets full of love,
Kate xx

And there you have it! Whether we meet in the pages of another book or in the comforting sphere of a coaching session, I look forward to being part of your continued journey towards empowerment and well-being.

Here's to fabulous you!

CHAPTER 32
Perimenopause Glossary of Terms

A

Abnormal Uterine Bleeding (AUB)

Bleeding from the uterus that varies from a woman's normal menstrual cycle, which might be more common during the perimenopause phase.

Adrenals

Glands located on top of each kidney that produce hormones including cortisol and adrenaline. They also produce a small amount of sex hormones, which can play a role in perimenopause.

Amenorrhoea

The absence of menstruation for an extended period, typically marking the onset of perimenopause when it lasts for twelve consecutive months.

Anal Incontinence

The inability to control bowel movements, which can sometimes occur as a result of changes or damage to the pelvic floor muscles during perimenopause.

Androgenetic Alopecia

A common form of hair loss in both men and women, often becoming more noticeable in women after perimenopause due to hormonal changes.

Androgens

A group of sex hormones, including testosterone, that are present in both men and women, but usually in higher amounts in men. During perimenopause, the balance of these hormones can change.

Andropause

Often referred to as "male menopause," it refers to the gradual decrease of testosterone levels in men as they age.

Antidepressants

Medications used to treat depression, which can sometimes be prescribed to manage mood swings and depression associated with menopause.

Antimüllerian Hormone (AMH)

A hormone produced by ovarian follicles. Low levels can indicate reduced ovarian reserve, which might be a sign of impending perimenopause.

Anxiety

A mental health condition characterised by persistent, excessive worry, which can sometimes be exacerbated during perimenopause.

Aromatase Inhibitors

Medications that block the enzyme aromatase, which converts androgens into oestrogens, sometimes used in the treatment of hormone-sensitive cancers and conditions.

Arthritis

A condition characterised by inflammation of the joints, which can sometimes worsen during perimenopause due to changes in hormone levels.

B

Belly Breathing

A type of deep breathing where the belly expands during inhalation, used as a relaxation technique to manage stress and anxiety, which can be beneficial during perimenopause.

Bilateral Oophorectomy

The surgical removal of both ovaries, which induces perimenopause as it halts the production of many female hormones.

Bio-identical Hormones/Body-Identical Hormones

Hormones that have the same chemical structure as those naturally produced by the body, often used in hormone replacement therapy during perimenopause.

Bladder Prolapse

A condition where the bladder descends into the vagina due to weakened pelvic floor muscles, which can occur during perimenopause.

Bone Mineral Density (BMD) or Bone Density

A measurement of the amount of minerals (calcium and phosphorus) contained in a certain volume of bone, used to diagnose osteoporosis, a condition more common after menopause.

BRCA1 and BRCA2 Genes

Genes that produce tumour suppressor proteins; mutations in these genes increase the risk of breast and ovarian cancer, and women with these mutations may undergo perimenopause earlier due to surgical removal of ovaries.

C

Cardiovascular Disease (CVD)

A class of diseases that involve the heart and blood vessels, the risk of which can increase post-menopause.

Cervix

The lower, narrow end of the uterus that connects the uterus to the vagina. It can be affected by hormonal changes during perimenopause.

Cholesterol

A waxy, fat-like substance found in all cells of the body, levels of which can change during perimenopause, potentially increasing the risk of heart disease.

Chronic Condition

A long-lasting health condition that may not have a cure, several of which can be influenced by perimenopause, including cardiovascular diseases and osteoporosis.

Climacteric

The phase in a woman's life during which she transitions from reproductive age to non-reproductive age, encompassing both perimenopause and post-menopause.

Cognitive Changes

Changes in memory or cognitive function, which some women experience during perimenopause.

Cognitive Function

The mental processes that allow us to carry out tasks, which can sometimes be affected during perimenopause, potentially leading to memory issues or difficulty concentrating.

Compounded Bioidentical Hormones

Custom-made hormones prepared by a pharmacist to be bi-oidentical to a person's natural hormones, used in hormone therapy during perimenopause.

Continuous Combination Therapy

A type of hormone therapy often used during menopause, where a combination of oestrogen and progestin are taken continuously to manage symptoms.

Custom-Compounded Hormones

Hormones custom-prepared to suit individual needs, often used in bioidentical hormone therapy for perimenopause.

Cystectomy

Surgical removal of an ovarian cyst, frequently performed with a minimally invasive technique called laparoscopy ("keyhole surgery").

Cystitis

Inflammation of the bladder, which can occur more frequently in post-menopausal women due to changes in the urinary tract.

D

Deep Vein Thrombosis (DVT)

A blood clot that forms in a deep vein, usually in the leg. The risk can be increased with certain types of hormone therapy used during perimenopause.

Dehydroepiandrosterone (DHEA)

A hormone produced by the adrenals that can be converted into oestrogen and testosterone. Its levels decline with age, and it is sometimes used in supplemental form during perimenopause.

DEXA Scan

A type of X-ray that measures bone mineral density, used to diagnose osteoporosis, which is more common in post-menopausal women.

Dilator

A medical device used to expand the vaginal opening and treat vaginal atrophy, a condition that can occur during perimenopause due to decreased oestrogen levels.

Dyspareunia

Painful intercourse, often resulting from vaginal dryness or atrophy, which can be a symptom of perimenopause.

E

Early Perimenopause/Menopause

The onset of menopause before the age of 45, which can occur naturally or as a result of medical interventions such as chemotherapy or surgery.

Early Ovarian Ageing

A condition where the ovaries age faster than normal, potentially leading to earlier onset of perimenopause/menopause

Endocrinology

The study of the endocrine system, which includes the glands and hormones in the body, and plays a significant role in perimenopause.

Endometrial Atrophy

Thinning of the lining of the uterus, often occurring as a result of decreased oestrogen levels during perimenopause.

Estrogen

Another spelling of the word oestrogen. A group of hormones responsible for the development of female sexual characteristics and the regulation of the menstrual cycle. Its levels fluctuate and decrease during perimenopause.

F

Follicle Stimulating Hormone (FSH)

A hormone that stimulates the growth of ovarian follicles. Its levels increase significantly as a woman approaches perimenopause.

FSH Test

A blood test that measures the level of follicle-stimulating hormone, which increases significantly as a woman approaches perimenopause.

G

Genitourinary

Pertaining to the genital and urinary systems. Menopause can affect the genito-urinary system, leading to symptoms like urinary incontinence and vaginal dryness.

Gynaecology

The medical practice specialising in the health of the female reproductive systems and the breasts.

H

Hormone Therapy (HRT)

Treatment involving the administration of hormones, typically oestrogen and/or progesterone, to alleviate symptoms of perimenopause.

Hot Flashes/Flushes

Sudden feelings of heat, typically affecting the face, neck, and chest, often accompanied by sweating and followed by chills, common during perimenopause.

Hysterectomy

A surgical procedure to remove the uterus, which may induce perimenopause if the ovaries are also removed.

I

Inflammation

A protective response by the body to injury or infection, which can be exacerbated during menopause, potentially contributing to development of chronic conditions.

Insomnia

Difficulty falling asleep or staying asleep, a common symptom experienced during perimenopause due to hormonal fluctuations.

Isoflavones

A type of phytoestrogen found in plants such as soy, sometimes used as a supplement to alleviate perimenopausal symptoms.

L

Libido

Sexual desire, which can fluctuate or decrease during perimenopause due to hormonal changes.

Lichen Sclerosis

A skin condition that affects the genital and anal areas, causing white patches and thinning skin. It is more common in post-menopausal women.

Luteinising Hormone (LH)

A hormone involved in the menstrual cycle, which sees increased levels during perimenopause.

M

Medical Menopause

Menopause that occurs as a result of medical interventions such as chemotherapy or surgery, rather than natural aging processes.

Menopause

The time in a woman's life when she stops having menstrual periods for twelve consecutive months, marking the end of her reproductive years, usually occurring between the ages of 45 and 55.

Menorrhagia

Excessive menstrual bleeding, which can sometimes occur during perimenopause as menstrual cycles become irregular.

Metabolic Syndrome

A cluster of conditions including increased blood pressure, high blood sugar, excess body fat around the waist, and abnormal cholesterol levels, which can be associated with increased risk of heart disease and is often more prevalent post-menopause.

Micronised Progesterone

A form of progesterone used in hormone therapy that is chemically identical to the progesterone produced by the ovaries, often used during perimenopause to manage symptoms.

Mirena Coil

A type of intrauterine device (IUD) that releases a small amount of progestin hormone into the uterus, sometimes used to manage menopausal symptoms.

N

NICE Guidelines

Guidelines issued by the National Institute for Health and Care Excellence in the UK, offering evidence-based recommendations on healthcare, including the management of perimenopause.

O

Oestrogen

A group of hormones responsible for the development and regulation of the female reproductive system, the levels of which decline during perimenopause.

Oestrogen Gel

A type of hormone therapy where oestrogen is administered through the skin via a gel, used to manage symptoms of perimenopause.

Oestrogen Patch

A type of hormone therapy where oestrogen is administered through the skin via a patch, used to manage symptoms of perimenopause.

Oestrogen Pessary

A vaginal suppository containing oestrogen, used to treat vaginal atrophy and dryness associated with perimenopause.

Oestrogen Tablets

Oral tablets containing oestrogen, used in hormone therapy to manage symptoms of perimenopause.

Oophorectomy

The surgical removal of one or both ovaries, which induces menopause by halting the production of many female hormones.

Osteoporosis

A condition characterised by weak and brittle bones, which can be exacerbated by the decrease in oestrogen levels during perimenopause.

P

Palpitations

Unpleasant sensations of irregular or forceful beating of the heart, which can sometimes be a symptom of perimenopause.

Pelvic Floor

A group of muscles that support the pelvic organs. These muscles can weaken during perimenopause, leading to issues such as urinary incontinence.

Phytoestrogens

Plant-derived compounds with estrogenic activity, sometimes used as supplements to manage perimenopausal symptoms.

Post-Menopause

The period of time after a woman has experienced twelve
consecutive months without a menstrual period, marking
the end of menopause.

Premature Menopause

Menopause that occurs before the age of 40, either naturally
or due to medical interventions.

Premature Ovarian Insufficiency

A condition where the ovaries lose function before the age
of 40, leading to early perimenopause.

Progesterone Tablets

Oral tablets containing progesterone, used in hormone therapy to manage symptoms of perimenopause, often in combination with oestrogen.

Psychosexual

Pertaining to the psychological aspects of sexual activity,
which can be affected during perimenopause due to symptoms like vaginal dryness or decreased libido.

R

Resistance Training

A type of physical exercise that involves opposing forces,
such as weightlifting. It can help to build muscle mass and
bone density, which can be beneficial during perimenopause.

Restless Legs Syndrome

A condition characterised by an uncontrollable urge to move the legs, often occurring in the evening or at night. It can sometimes be exacerbated during perimenopause.

S

Sequential Hormone Therapy

A type of hormone therapy often used during perimenopause, where different hormones are taken at different times of the menstrual cycle to manage symptoms.

Sexual Health

An important aspect of overall health, which can be affected during perimenopause due to changes in libido, vaginal dryness, etc.

Smear Test

Also known as a Pap smear, it is a procedure to test for cervical cancer in women by collecting cells from the cervix, which should continue to be regularly performed post-menopause.

Square Breathing

A breathing technique used to reduce stress and anxiety, involving inhaling, holding the breath, exhaling, and holding the breath again, all for equal counts, which can be beneficial during perimenopause.

Stress Incontinence

Involuntary leakage of urine during physical activity or coughing, sneezing, etc., which can occur due to weakened pelvic floor muscles during perimenopause.

Surgical Menopause

Menopause that occurs as a result of surgery to remove the ovaries or uterus, leading to a sudden drop in hormone levels.

T

Transdermal

Through the skin, refers to the administration of medications (like hormone therapy) through the skin via patches or gels, which can be used during perimenopause.

Thyroid Disorders

Disorders affecting the thyroid gland, which can sometimes mimic or exacerbate menopausal symptoms, as they also involve hormonal imbalances.

Triggers

Factors that can exacerbate menopausal symptoms, such as stress, alcohol, spicy foods, or smoking.

V

Vaginal Atrophy

Thinning, drying, and inflammation of the vaginal walls due to a decrease in oestrogen, often occurring during perimenopause.

Vaginal Rejuvenation

A general term for a variety of surgical and non-surgical procedures aimed at restoring or improving the aesthetic or functional aspects of the vaginal area, which some women may pursue during or after perimenopause.

Vasomotor Symptoms

Symptoms such as hot flashes and night sweats, which are caused by changes in the body's temperature regulation, common during perimenopause.

Vitamin D

A vitamin essential for bone health, which can be particularly important during perimenopause to prevent bone loss and osteoporosis.

Vulva

The external part of the female genitals, which can be affected by changes during perimenopause, including dryness and atrophy.

W

Weight Gain

An increase in body weight, which is common during perimenopause due to changes in hormones affecting metabolism and body composition.

Well Woman Check

A comprehensive health check for women, including screening for diseases and conditions that are more common or can be more serious in women, sometimes focusing on menopausal health.

Y

Yam Extract

A natural substance extracted from yams, sometimes used as a component in bioidentical hormone replacement therapy, although its effectiveness is debated.

Yearly Check-Up

> An annual health check-up to monitor one's health status and screen for potential issues, including assessments relevant to perimenopause such as bone density tests and cholesterol checks.

Yoga

> A physical, mental, and spiritual practice that can help manage menopausal symptoms by reducing stress, improving flexibility, and increasing muscle strength.

CHAPTER 33
Useful Resources

Support Groups and Forums

Perimenopause with Kate Grosvenor: My Facebook support group that you are most welcome to join. It offers support, advice, coaching, etc. and is a place where you can ask questions and join in discussions. You can go to this link or scan the QR code below. https://www.facebook.com/groups/perimenopausewithkategrosvenor/

Menopause Support Network: A UK-based group offering community support and expert advice. https://menopausesupport.co.uk

Products

For bamboo bedding, underwear, and nightwear you can visit my collection at:www.kategrosvenorlifestyle.com

For natural deodorants, the best when I've found personally is from https://saltoftheearthnatural.com

Aromatherapy oils and toxic-free beauty and cleaning products, please see www.kategrosvenorlifestyle.com

Tea Pigs herbal teas are my absolute fave. They are made from using as much of the whole natural plant as possible and come in plastic-free and compostable tea bags. https://www.teapigs.co.uk

Videos

Cocoa Breaths: this is a great video on my YouTube channel for learning a simple and memorable breathing technique to feel calmer and less anxious instantly. https://youtu.be/szexkGIXG9Q?si=4JnN9oTDscrQMRSm

Professional Resources

National Institute for Health and Care Excellence (NICE) Guidelines: Provides evidence-based best practice advice, particularly useful if you're in the UK. https://www.nice.org.uk/guidance/ng23/chapter/recommendations

The North American Menopause Society: A hub for healthcare providers and the public offering a wide range of educational resources. https://www.menopause.org

The British Menopause Society (BMS) new Menopause Practice Standards for Health Care Professionals: https://thebms.org.uk/wp-content/uploads/2022/07/BMS-Menopause-Practice-Standards-JULY2022-01D.pdf

INDEX

Abdominal Fat, 91

Abdominal Pain, 109

Acupuncture, 77, 80, 123, 135, 189

Allergies, 36, 216

Androgen Dominance, 251

Anxiety, 29, 82, 124, 130, 168, 279, 326

Apple Cider Vinegar, 89, 108

Arianna Huffington, 95

Bacteria, 95

Bloating, 30, 92

Brain fog, 29

Breast Soreness/Tenderness, 210

Breast Swelling, 212

Butterbur, 77

Caffeine, 122, 133, 166, 174, 213, 218, 226, 287

Calm, 48, 131

Chamomile, 108, 110, 126, 129, 131, 134, 143, 146, 179, 293

Chest Pain, 207

Children, 139

Chronic Stress, 128, 171

Cinnamon, 89

Clumsiness, 201

Cognitive Behavioural Therapy (CBT), 126, 131, 296

Cold Flashes, 189

Comparititis, 310

Concentration, 63

Constipation, 53

Cortisol, 24, 46

Couples Therapy, 138

DAO, 82, 83

Depression, 29, 126, 281, 283

DHEA, 249, 330

Diarrhoea, 31, 107

Digestive Problems, 105

Dizzy Spells, 192

Dry Eyes, 220

Eleanor Roosevelt, 17, 28, 68

Emotional Eating, 88, 100, 104, 309

Emotional Numbness, 128

Emotional Vulnerability, 295

Employers and Co-Workers, 145

Environmental Awareness, 267

Exercise, 25, 54, 58, 63, 79, 88, 91, 99, 102, 106, 109, 122, 125, 127, 129, 131, 132, 134, 138, 166,

173, 177, 182, 208, 209, 214,
215, 218, 222, 227, 230, 266,
280, 281, 284, 290, 291, 297,
300, 307
Fear of Change, 303
Feverfew, 76
Flaxseed, 55, 274
Follicle Stimulating Hormone
(FSH), 331
Food Cravings, 103
Friends, 129, 141, 295
Frozen Shoulder, 180
Ginger, 77, 108, 110, 177, 190,
193, 196, 198
Ginkgo Biloba, 67
Green Tea, 89
Gut Dysbiosis, 94
Gut Health, 53
Hair, 34, 150
Headaches, 32, 72, 80, 82
Heart Health, 51
History of, 63, 257
Honest Conversations, 142
Hormone Replacement
Therapy, 53, 58, 71, 75, 158
Hot Flushes/Flashes, 184
Hydration, 65, 68, 70, 73, 77, 93,
106, 107, 116, 155, 156, 166,
188, 210, 213, 220, 222
Imposter Syndrome, 305, 306,
307
In the USA, 260
Infections, 32, 222

Insomnia, 30, 159, 163, 164, 165,
285, 287, 332
Insulin Resistance, 88, 91
Irritability, 29, 132, 133, 137, 144,
290
Isolation, 128, 142
Itchy Ears, 196
Joint Pain, 176
Lack of Motivation, 302
Lavender, 77, 126, 129, 133, 140,
146, 179
Learning, 69, 129
Lewis, 71
Localised Oestrogen, 252, 253
Low self-esteem, 298, 300
Luteinising Hormone, 333
Luteinising Hormone (LH), 333
Maca Root, 118, 139, 316
Magnesium, 76, 126, 131, 133,
179, 188, 215, 316
Mary Wollstonecraft, 82
Maya Angelou, 26, 65, 97
Meal box services, 276
Memory, 29, 61, 65
Menstrual Cycle, 33
Migraines, 32, 74
Mindfulness, 25, 47, 63, 67, 75,
89, 104, 123, 125, 127, 129, 134,
144, 163, 166, 174, 186, 194,
200, 201, 203, 207, 214, 215,
219, 220, 223, 227, 230, 279,
282, 285, 286, 291, 292, 299,
301, 308, 309

Mirena Coil, 242, 243, 246, 334

Mood swings, 16, 30, 133, 135, 283

Muscle Aches, 182

Muscle Tension, 178

National Institute for Health and Care Excellence (NICE), 38, 39, 183, 263, 342

Nausea, 31, 198

Night Sweats, 170, 187

Nutrition, 49, 66, 83, 86, 95, 99, 102, 121, 122, 145, 154, 166, 172, 183, 220, 228, 280, 287

Oestrobolome, 85, 86, 87

Oestrogen, 16, 18, 62, 63, 83, 86, 90, 115, 116, 134, 151, 176, 177, 204, 206, 235, 236, 237, 242, 281, 334, 335

Omega-3, 67, 79, 89, 126, 128, 133, 135, 138, 177, 221, 274, 284, 317

Osteoporosis, 35, 56, 335

Panic Attacks/Disorder, 130

Parents, 143

Passionflower, 126, 131

Peppermint, 76, 108, 110, 198

Perimenopause, 1, 2, 3, 5, 6, 11, 13, 15, 27, 36, 37, 38, 42, 67, 68, 69, 72, 74, 78, 88, 96, 101, 107, 109, 116, 118, 121, 123, 126, 133, 134, 151, 157, 165, 169, 170, 171, 174, 226, 233, 255, 259, 261, 262, 263, 266, 268, 272, 280, 297, 299, 304, 306, 313, 322, 325, 330, 341

Phantom Smells, 206

Phytoestrogens, 186, 270, 271, 274, 336

POI, 16, 41, 42

Probiotics, 95, 108, 224, 317

Procrastination, 304

Progesterone, 20, 46, 242, 243, 247, 334, 336

Relationships, 54

Restless Legs Syndrome, 217, 337

Restlessness, 35, 230

Risk Factors, 239

Rosemary Essential Oil, 67

Scheduled Intimacy, 138

Serotonin, 47, 48

Shortness of Breath, 208

Skin Care, 151, 157

Sleep, 16, 54, 66, 67, 70, 76, 88, 96, 101, 123, 132, 146, 157, 159, 161, 162, 163, 165, 166, 168, 170, 174, 175, 189, 223, 230, 231, 267, 281, 285, 286, 290

Slow Cooker, 274, 276

St John's Wort, 127, 133

Stress, 24, 32, 45, 54, 67, 73, 75, 78, 83, 88, 89, 92, 93, 102, 105, 106, 107, 110, 111, 116, 122, 132, 145, 157, 168, 174, 179, 181, 185, 194, 198, 199, 201, 202, 206, 208, 214, 217, 223, 227, 291, 292, 337

Stress Incontinence, 32, 111, 337

Supplements, 59, 79, 122, 126,
145, 157, 179, 188, 215, 218, 223,
225, 271, 272, 313

Susceptibility, 222

Symptoms, 16, 24, 27, 35, 38, 81,
127, 174, 251, 268, 272, 339

Testosterone, 21, 117, 250, 251,
252

Tinnitus, 34, 194

To test or not to test, 37

Urinary Problems, 32

Vaginal atrophy, 32, 115, 252

Vaginal dryness, 32, 114, 116

Valerian Root, 129, 131, 140

Vertigo, 34, 195

Virginia Woolf, 124

Vitamin D, 128, 138, 173, 319, 339

Walking, 53

Weight Gain, 30, 87, 177, 339

Printed in Great Britain
by Amazon

30204453R00192